Yes Women Lift

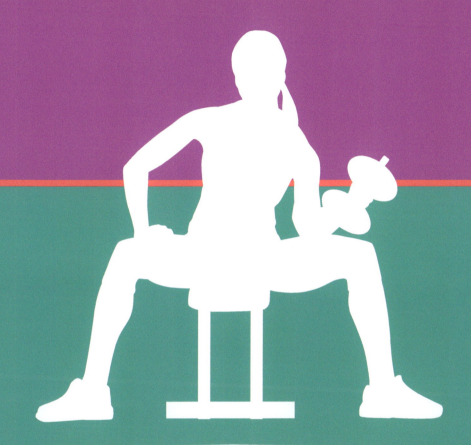

FEEL FIT, EMPOWERED & UNSTOPPABLE

DISCLAIMER

Every effort has been made to make all publications and products sold through this site or through phone and mail as complete and accurate as possible. However, there may be mistakes both typographical and in content. Therefore, this text should be used only as a general guide and not as the ultimate reference source.

The information presented in this publication is not intended as specific medical advice and is not a substitute for professional medical treatment or diagnosis.

The contents of this publication, including articles, graphics, images, and all other material, are for your private use and informational purposes only. If you have a medical emergency, do not rely on the content to treat your condition; call your doctor or go to a hospital immediately. The content is not intended to be professional medical advice, diagnosis, or treatment.

Always seek the advice of your physician or other qualified health professional with any questions you may have regarding any medical concerns or conditions.

Reliance on the content or any other information provided by Laticia Jackson or any of her employees, agents, authors or others providing content to this book is solely at your own risk. The content is provided on an "as is" basis.

If at any time during exercise you feel faint, shortness of breath or dizziness, stop activity and seek medical attention.

Yes Women Lift!

Published in arrangement with

www.laticiaactionjackson.com

By

Laticia "Action" Jackson

Masters of Public Health (M.P.H.)

Fitness Expert /B.S. Exercise Science/C.P.T.

Certified Lifestyle and Weight Management Specialist

Certified Senior Weight Loss Counselor

3-Time N.P.C. Fitness Champion

I.F.B.B. Fitness Professional and 2008 Fitness Olympian

Fitness Images by Jiame Rivera

Jar Studio.com

Visit our website at

www.laticiaactionjackson.com

TESTIMONIALS

"Laticia "Action" Jackson is a student of the game and a master of her craft."

Daryl Haley ~ Retired N.F.L New England Patriots

"Laticia Jackson is a fitness inspiration who walks the walk.

Follow her lead and you're sure to change your body for the better."

Brad Schoenfeld, MS, CSCS ~ Author: Women's Home Workout Bible

---

"Undeniably the best fitness trainer I have ever had the privilege to interview or work with. She pushes you to be your best. Not only physically- and believe me she's tough. But internally which gives you the permission to be your best- mind, body and spirit!"

Mark Mathis ~ CW31 Good Day Sacramento

"One Dynamic Lady... whose passion to succeed and make a difference has made her dynamic in all areas of her life."

Mike Lackner ~ Body Fitness-UK

"Every workout was earnest, extremely enjoyable and tailored to my personal needs allowing me to reach my maximum physical fitness level. Laticia was inspirational, motivating and I highly endorse her as a physical fitness trainer for anyone and everyone."

Lloyd C. ~ Colonel U.S.A.F., Dayton Ohio

"Working with Laticia as my personal trainer has been an empowering experience. She teaches your mind new fitness concepts and encourages your inner self to embrace and love the healthy person you are destined to be."

Sandra H. ~ California Police Dept., Sacramento, CA

Table of Contents

Dedication

This book is dedicated to the woman who desires to feel FIT, EMPOWERED and UNSTOPPABLE! Fit, empowered and unstoppable is how I feel each time I pick up a dumbbell, and it is my desire that you will feel the same way too! I know that the gym can be an intimidating environment for many women, however, this book will give you the knowledge and confidence you need to start using weight lifting as a tool to tone and strengthen your body, increase your confidence, and safely push your body further than you ever have before.

This book is not about teaching you how to get the perfect body. It's about teaching you how to get into the best shape of your life, while feeling great about your body! The benefits of weight training are simply too many to keep them all to myself. Weight training promotes increased calorie burn, stronger bones, stronger muscles to perform everyday tasks, and even burning more calories while you sleep. Yes, this all happens when you build lean, strong muscles!

Let me help you say goodbye to gym intimidation, and hello to a fit, empowered and unstoppable you!

LOVE ACTION JACKSON

STAY FIT, STAY TRUE,

STAY YOU!

Acknowledgments

First and most importantly, I would like to thank my Creator for entrusting me with this vision. I am forever grateful for the gifts you have given me. May I always live a life that is pleasing and honorable in your sight. I love you and will always need you. You are amazing.

Mom, there are not enough words in the dictionary to describe how much I love you. Regardless of what life has brought my way, you have always been there to love me through my trials. A day without you is comparable to a day without the sun. You are my light and my best friend. I pray that one day I will be a great mother just like you. I miss our girl nights out and spending quality time with you.

Dad, you have always been a silent strength in my life. I have inherited your tremendous work ethic and it has paid off in so many ways. You are a man of great character and integrity and I pray to one day marry a man with your morals and values. I look forward to our relationship growing. It's great to find out who I get my long arms from!

Yolanda, I would like to thank you for always being there for me. You are always just a call away. You are officially my human resource person. Your strength as a soldier, mother, sister, wife and friend is encouraging. May God give you all the desires of your heart and much more. I pray you learn to laugh more often; you know I do enough laughing for the both of us. You are a great big sister and I love you.

Shanta, we have been friends for as long as I can remember. Even though you have left me outside in the cold to get a donut, I will always love you. You are the true image of a wife and mother. You are selfless and I admire that about you. Your constant prayers, love and encouragement is priceless. You have a special place in my heart. I love you butterfly. Thanks for letting me be your little sister.

To MKS, you have taught me the true meaning of unconditional love and I love you more and more each day. You're a great man of integrity and I treasure the laughter we share. You definitely have all of my heart and I look forward to our future together!

To my nieces and nephews, you bring so much joy to my life. It has been such a pleasure to be your auntie. Seeing each of you grow up brings joy to my heart. I love each of you.

To my brother-in-laws, thanks for loving my sisters and being great men.

LET YOUR FITNESS JOURNEY BEGIN!

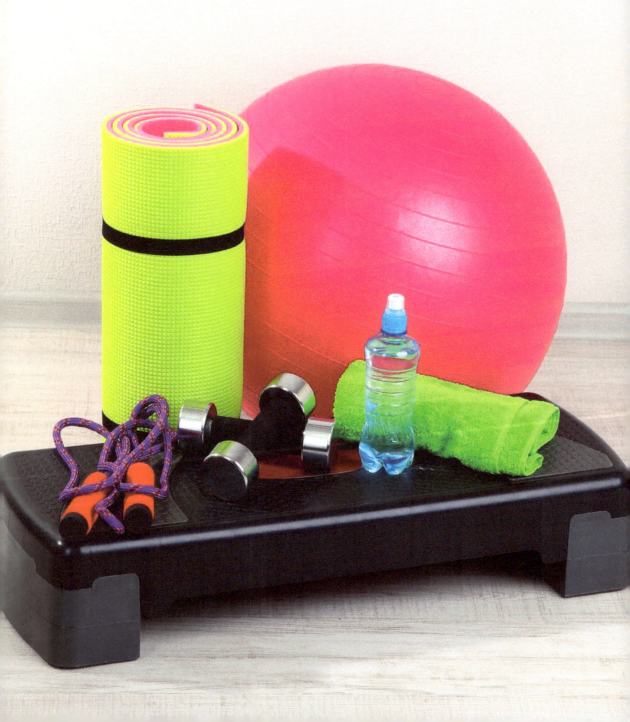

Introduction

As a 2008 Fitness Olympian and 3-Time NPC Fitness Champion, I have built my career on having a strong and fit body. I have stood on stages performing one-armed push-ups and other strength moves that helped propel my fitness career to the highest level one can achieve-- the Fitness Olympia, where I was ranked 8th in the world in 2008.

Accomplishing this level of athletic success required a great deal of training in the gym. Yes, in the gym. That smelly place where many women DON'T want to venture!

In fact, if I logged all the hours I spent in the gym over the last 15 years, they would be too numerous to count. I've had some of my most memorable experiences and have built some of my most precious friendships in this setting.

However as I approached my 30's and began to take more notice of my surroundings in the gym, I began to realize that there were few women who actually used the weight room.

I observed many women spending their gym time either in the cardiovascular area or in fitness classes such as Zumba, Kick Boxing or Pilates.

Although these activities can be great workouts, they alone cannot transform a woman's body the way weight training can.

I WANTED TO KNOW WHY!

MY CURIOSITY BEGAN to get the best of me, so I started asking women about their exercise habits and preferences.

I wanted to learn whether other women were interested in lifting weights and, if they were, what barriers were standing in the way of them actually doing it.

The women I spoke to had various reasons for shying away from weight training, such as, "I don't want to look manly" or, "I want to lose body fat first and then lift weights," but the most repeated reason I encountered was: "I don't know what to do and I feel intimidated."

GREAT FEEDBACK

GATHERING THIS INFORMATION helped me understand the challenges and misinformation women face when considering weight training. I realized that I could use my 15 years of experience to help women tackle these obstacles and share the feelings of empowerment, strength, and health that weight training has helped me to enjoy.

Therefore in the following pages I will outline misconceptions about women and weight training, how to identify your body type and assess your current fitness level, how to set fitness training goals based on your fitness assessment results, how to lift weights based on your fitness skill level, and how to understand spoken and unspoken gym rules with gym girls' etiquette.

Are you excited?

If you are, let the reading begin!

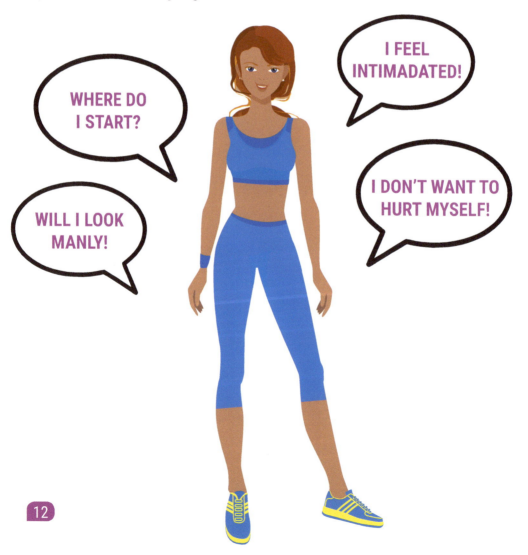

PART 1

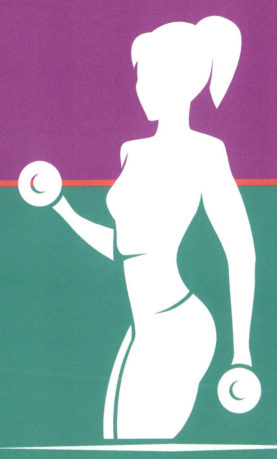

DESTINATION FIT

I Don't Want to Look Like a Man!

Have you ever thought about starting a weight lifting or resistance training fitness program, but you were afraid that building muscle would cause you to appear less feminine, or "manly"? If this is you, you are not alone!

For years, women have been led to believe that if they lift weights then they will become muscular and manly looking.

Have you bought into this myth?

Allow me to put this misconception to rest, and explain why you will not appear manly if and when you add weight lifting to your fitness program.

YOU WON'T LOOK LIKE A MAN

WOMEN NATURALLY HAVE lower levels of a masculine hormone called testoterone. Testosterone is the hormone that gives men their manly features such as facial hair, deep voices and dense muscle tissues.

Most women posses small amounts of this hormone in their bodies, therefore they do not produce large manly muscles from lifting weights. Therefore if or when you see women with large muscles, typically they are athletes or female bodybuilders who intentionally use heavy weight to progressively build their muscles. Their muscular growth is builit to perform at optimal levels for their particular sport or built to perform on the bodybuilding stage. Therefore the chances of a women getting bulky muscles from lifting light to moderate amounts of weight is slim to none.

Now that we have put that myth to rest allow me to tell you about the many benefits of lifting weights.

THE BENEFITS ARE MANY!

ACCORDING TO THE American College of Sports Medicine (ACSM), weight training should be an intergral part of an healthy adults fitness training program. Weight training can assist you in burning more body fat, buliding stronger bones, increasing your metabolism, and even burning calories while you rest!

And, as if those benefits alone aren't reason enough to incorporate weight training into your fitness regimen, there's more! Research has shown that weight training can boost one's self-esteem by increasing greater body satisfaction and increase mood enhancing chemicals!

LIFTING WEIGHTS IS EMPOWERING!

OVER THE LAST 15 years, I have been able to use resistance training to help me sculpt my body and become one of the world's top ranked athletes. When I lift weights I feel powerful and unstoppable!

I'm completely mindful that it may not be your goal to become an athlete, but I do want to encourage you to try lifting weights, because I know you'll enjoy feeling as empowered as I do.

It is my hope that by giving you the knowledge that you can transform the shape of your body, create stronger bones and feel empowered by your own strength, you will either start or continuing lifting weights!

DON'T DO IT ALONE

IF YOU FEEL intimated by starting a weight training program, hire a personal trainer for a few sessions and allow him or her to teach you the proper way to lift weights. At first you may feel like a fish out of water, but I am confident that once you see the results and you begin to challenge your mind to push your body harder than you have ever pushed before, you won't be able to put the weights down.

I have coached too many women throughout this process to list them all, however, if you trust that I have your best interest at heart, you will become addicted to lifting weights – in a good way, of course – and you will achieve excellent results.

THE EMPOWERMENT IS ENDLESS

EACH TIME I leave a lifting session, I feel more and more empowered, and excited for the next time. These feelings have kept me going back to the gym for over 15 years and I've NEVER regretted a workout!

I know you will feel the same way!

Are you ready to learn how to start the process?

If you are, let the reading continue.

IT'S TIME TO FEEL FIT & EMPOWERED

Where Do You Begin?

For many women, the thought of beginning a fitness-training program is an exciting life changing adventure, but often, this excitement gets replaced with frustration and confusion.

The feeling of frustration is often the result of not knowing where or how to start their fitness-training program.

With so many books on fitness, some women are left feeling overwhelmed, confused and discouraged.

Have you ever felt this way?

If you have, your frustration is over. I am about to take you step-by-step and teach you how to get into the best shape of your life by incorporating lifting weights or what is known as resistance training!

Are you ready? Let's take the first step!

LET THE JOURNEY BEGIN

THE FIRST STEP to getting in shape is to discover your body type. Every woman's body type is unique therefore knowing your body type will provide you with an understanding of how your body responds to exercise and how to properly train.

Understanding your body type will hopefully help you from comparing your body to your girlfriends and other women.

Therefore, let's identify your body type.

STEP 1. DISCOVER YOUR BODY TYPE

DISCOVERING YOUR BODY type is an important step in creating an individualized fitness-training program to meet your individualized fitness goals. Having an understanding of your body type will help you set realistic goals and expectations and relieve you from trying to make your girlfriend's fitness program work for you.

They are three main body types, which include ectomorph (banana), mesomorph (apple or triangle) and endomorph (bell or pear). It is common for women to be a combination of two body types. Due to your individuality, it is important that you do not compare your body to other women. Your body may be smaller on top and larger on the bottom, or you may be larger on top and smaller on the bottom. Whatever your body type, you have your own unique structural foundation and your training should be tailored accordingly.

Below are descriptions of each body type and the recommended resistance and cardiovascular training. Read all descriptions and determine which is a realistic category for your body.

"YOUR BODY IS A MASTERPIECE AND YOU'RE THE ARTISTS!"

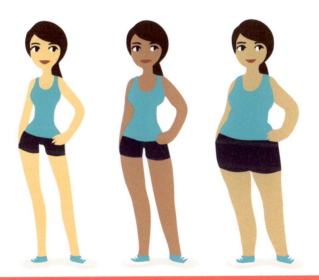

LET'S DISCOVER YOUR BODY TYPE

ECTOMORPH BODY TYPE

Body Description

Thin body structure, short torso, thin limbs and narrow feet and hands. Has difficulty putting on weight and does not carry a lot of muscle.

Unlike the mesomorph and the endomorph, the ectomorph is a person who has been skinny their entire life. It is not a result of a good diet or strict workout ethics. They are born with a superfast metabolism which allows their body to break food down at a higher rate. This gives them the "ability" to eat whatever they desire and not gain weight.

Resistance Training

The use of moderately light weights in combination with a repetition range of 12-15 can help tone the ectomorph body type. People with this body type may lack strength, therefore if strength is a goal, lifting heavier weight is required (15 pounds or more) to become stronger.

Cardiovascular Activity

Due to the high metabolism of this body type, performing an excessive amount of cardiovascular activity is not advantageous. Performing high amounts of cardio will prevent this body type from developing lean, toned muscles. Therefore performing 30 to 35 minutes of cardiovascular activities will help maintain lean muscle and not promote a stringy appearance and be sufficient to maintain cardiovascular health. Sufficient caloric intake is important to fuel this body type.

MESOMORPH BODY TYPE

Body Description

Naturally athletic, broad shoulders, narrow waist and the ability to gain muscle easily. Unlike the ectomorph, this body type doesn't have a problem gaining weight in the form of muscle or fat.

Resistance Training

Moderate to heavy weights can be used (depending on current fitness level) to maintain athletic build. A range of 8-15 repetitions with 3-4 sets per muscle group will help build dense muscle tissue without giving the bulky look. If you desire less muscle, incorporate lighter weight in conjunction with a repetition range of 15-20.

Cardiovascular Activity

Perform cardiovascular activities (running, cycling) at least 4 to 5 days per week for at least 45 minutes. Cardiovascular activity can be performed in an interval fashion (short bursts of high intensity activity, followed by lower intensities of recovery).

ENDOMORPH BODY TYPE

Body Description

Round, usually short in stature, carries a lot of body fat around mid- section and lower body. Slow metabolism and gains weight easily.

Resistance Training

Cardiovascular and resistance training is the key for this body type. Light to moderate weight with a repetition range of 12-15 with 3-4 sets per exercise will help tone and not build muscle. Performing activities in a circuit fashion is beneficial due to the constant state of movement throughout sets that will keep heart rate up which in return will burn more calories.

Cardiovascular Activity

Moderate to high intensity cardiovascular 45 minutes to 1 hour 4 to 5 days per week is recommended. Cardiovascular activities can be performed in an interval fashion (short bursts of high intensity activity, followed by lower intensities of recovery).

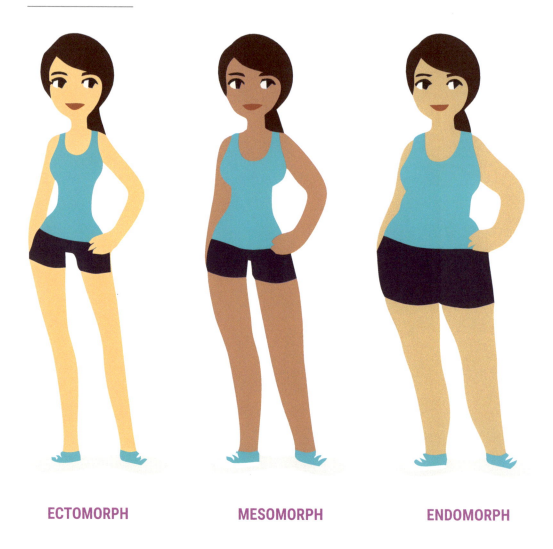

ECTOMORPH   **MESOMORPH**   **ENDOMORPH**

STEP 2. SET YOUR FITNESS GOALS

YOU HAVE DISCOVERED your body type, now it is time to learn how to set fitness training goals.

WHY IS IT IMPORTANT TO SET GOALS?

WHETHER IT IS financial, marital, spiritual or physical, goal setting is an important aspect of life that keeps you focused, motivated, action-oriented and accountable. In reference to setting fitness goals, your goals should be objective, measurable, short-term, long-term and challenging - yet realistic.

BE OBJECTIVE WITH YOUR GOALS

MAKING THE BROAD statement that you want to become fit is not concrete nor objective. You're definition of being fit needs narrowing down to a more specific or objective goal. Do you want to lose weight, gain lean muscle or improve your cardio-vascular conditioning? Whatever your goal, it needs to be defined. Once your goal is defined, you can begin taking the necessary steps required to reach your desired outcome.

MEASURE YOUR SUCCESS

GOALS NEED TO be measurable. How will you determine if you are making progress if you don't know where you started? One way to determine the success of any fit-ness-training program is to establish a baseline of measurements. These measure-ments could be your body fat percentage, amount of push-ups you can perform or how quickly you can run a specific distance. Every four to six weeks you can re-access this information to determine the progress you are making towards reaching your fitness goals.

TIME IS OF THE ESSENCE

SETTING A TIME frame to reach your goals is imperative to reaching your destination. You can set both short-term and long-term goals that will keep you focused and accountable.

Short-term goals are goals you want to accomplish within the next 3 to 6 months, whereas long-term goals can be accomplished within 6 months and beyond. If you are a procrastinator, setting short-term goals is very important to keep you focused and accountable. Deciding not to establish a time frame to accomplish your goal(s) threatens your chance of reaching your desired outcome.

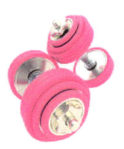

FIT JEWEL
Don't focus on your girlfriend's goals, establish your own. Your goals should be just as unique as you are!

SET CHALLENGING YET REALISTIC GOALS

FINALLY, GOALS NEED to be challenging, yet realistic. Setting unrealistic goals perpetuates the feeling of discouragement and failure. Failure of goal attainment isn't always based on a lack of effort on your part, rather a result of setting goals that were not realistically attainable. Challenge yourself, but be realistic with your expectations.

GUIDELINES FOR GOAL SETTING

- Goals should be measurable.
- Goals should be challenging, yet attainable.
- Set short-term and long-term goals.
- Goals should be specific and objective.

BENEFITS OF SETTING GOALS

- Greater sense of personal achievement
- Balanced life
- Increased motivation
- Improved self-confidence
- Better decision making
- Better focus
- Improved time management
- Over all self-improvement
- AND SUCCESS!

STEP 3. MEASURE AND ASSESS

YOU HAVE DISCOVERED your body type, have learned how to set fitness goals and now it's time to discuss the importance of measurements.

WHY ARE MEASUREMENTS IMPORTANT?

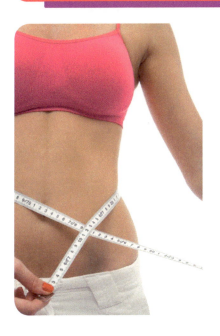

MEASUREMENTS ARE AN essential component to the success of your fitness program or weight loss program. Prior to starting any fitness or weight loss program, it is important to gather a baseline of information to determine a starting point and an ending point. How will you know if you're making progress towards your desired goal if you don't know where you started?

Baseline measurements can include your current weight, Body Mass Index (B.M.I), muscular endurance, flexibility and muscular strength testing. Gathering information from these sources can help you keep track of your results and every 4 to 6 weeks comparing your current results to your starting baseline measurements.

Below you will discover the most common methods used to gather baseline information.

METHODS OF MEASURING BODY COMPOSITION

WHEN YOU HEAR the words body composition, what do you think? Do you know what these words mean?

In the health and fitness world, these words are thrown around like a hot dog at a baseball game. These words are familiar to personal trainers and health care providers, but they may be foreign to you.

Body composition is a term used to describe the components that make up your body, such as lean mass, fat mass and water. One primary goal of any fitness or weight loss program is to decrease fat mass and increase lean mass. Don't worry, you won't get bulky and look manly from gaining lean and toned muscle mass.

It is important to decrease fat mass and increase lean muscle tissue for many health reasons. Fat mass such as visceral fat which surrounds the internal organs has been linked to various health concerns, such as diabetes, hypertension and some forms of cancer.

Therefore, in order to make improvements in your health (and not just your appearance), you need a fitness program that focuses on gaining lean, toned muscle while at the same time losing amounts of unwanted body fat.

SO HOW CAN YOU DETERMINE HOW MUCH BODY FAT AND LEAN MUSCLE MASS YOU HAVE?

THERE ARE SEVERAL different ways that are free and painless!

I know a lot of you cringe at the thought of getting your measurements done but no worries, in the end, it will benefit your health and you will look great.

I DON'T WANT TO KNOW MY NUMBERS!

IF YOU ARE one of those women who cringe at the thought of seeing measurements from your body, I want to put you at ease. These numbers don't define you; they just help to establish a starting point. I know - numbers, numbers and more numbers. You may be asking "Do I have to?" My answer is, "YES."

I promise you, the process will be done quickly and it's painless.

We are now going to discuss the three most common and inexpensive ways to get your body composition measurements done.

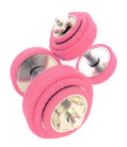

FIT JEWEL
You'll never know how far you've come,
if you don't know where you started.

FAT CALIPERS

WHAT IS A fat caliper and how does it work?

A fat caliper is a small non-expensive prong-like tool used to measure subcutaneous (underneath skin) body fat. The tester will have you stand in an upright position with arms out to your side. He or she will ask to touch your right arm and then proceed to mark designated anatomical locations (body) with a marker. The tester will then take their index finger and thumb and grasp at least 2 inches of your skin. The caliper will slightly grab your skin and then be released. This is a painless process that will take a few minutes to complete.

Once each spot has been located and measured, data (numbers) from the measurements are plugged into an equation to determine your percentage of body fat. Fat caliper measurements are not exact measurements, but provide you with a baseline of numbers to establish your current state of fat mass.

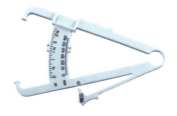

In order to have consistency with your measurements, have the same person administer your testing. Although each tester is required to use the same anatomical (body) locations, some testers measure differently. This difference could cause a slight variation in your numbers. You can visit your local gym or wellness center and request to have this test done for a required fee.

Below is a list of the most common anatomical locations used for measurements.

ANATOMICAL MEASURING LOCATIONS

- Triceps (back of arm)
- Supra iliac (top of hip bone)
- Sub-scapula (beneath shoulder blade)
- Biceps (middle of arm between shoulder and elbow)
- Midaxiallary- below armpit
- Subscapula-below shoulder blade
- Thigh - midway between top of hip and knee

GIRTH MEASUREMENTS

WHAT IS A GIRTH MEASUREMENT?

A girth measurement is a measurement that records the distance around a body part. Using this method is a non-expensive and convenient way to measure your body circumference and can be done by yourself or a trained professional. Girth measurements are sometimes used as a measure of body fat, but are not a valid predictor of this, however, can be used to measure proportionality.

HOW ARE GIRTH MEASUREMENTS TAKEN?

The only tool required to take your girth measurements is a flexible measuring tape. The person administering these measurements will use specified anatomical locations. To ensure as much accuracy as possible, the person administering the test should make sure measuring tape isn't positioned too tight or too loose and the tape is placed in a horizontal position.

Having the tape too tight or too loose will not give you accurate measurements. Once data is collected, the administrator will use a formula to give you a total for each of your measurements. If you do not have someone to do your measurements for you, the process is simple enough to do the measurements on your own. If you are measuring yourself, once you gather your numbers write them down in your journal and every 4-6 weeks compare your numbers to see if they are changing. It is important to remember if you are building muscle tissue some numbers may increase. That is expected so do not be alarmed.

WHERE DO YOU TAKE YOUR GIRTH MEASUREMENTS?

There are several different places to take your measurements

- **Bust:** measure all the way around your bust and back starting at the nipple line.

- **Waist:** measure at the smallest point around your mid- section two inches above your navel.

- **Thigh:** measure at the largest part of thigh, midway between hip and knee bone.

- **Calf muscle:** measure largest part midway between knee cap and ankle.

- **Arm:** measure the largest part of arm midway between shoulder joint and elbow.

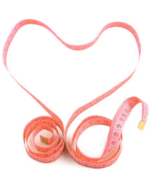

- **Hips:** measure the largest part of your buttocks, place tape on thighs and measure all the way around largest part of hips.

WEIGHT SCALE

USING A WEIGHT scale is a cheap and convenient way to track your weight loss or gain. You can order an inexpensive scale online or you may visit your neighborhood Wal-Mart or Walgreens to purchase a more advanced scale that is capable of recording your body fat percentage and lean muscle mass. These advanced scales are more costly, but a great investment.

Although using a weight scale is a quick and convenient way to track your weight loss or gain, if not used in moderation, this method could lead to counterproductive behaviors.

Weighing yourself too often may discourage and distract you. It is important to remember that your body changes on a daily basis, and as a result your numbers may not always be consistent. Therefore, do not depend solely on the scale to dictate your progress. Although not recommended, if you decide to weigh yourself daily, do it early in the morning at the same time on a regular basis prior to eating or drinking anything - this is your true bodyweight.

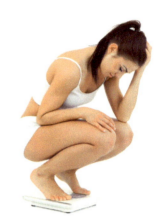

 Do not weigh yourself more than once a week. Healthy weight loss is a pound to two pounds per week. If you have a considerable amount of weight to lose (100lbs or more), you may lose more in beginning but will eventually tapper off. Eventually your body will stop shedding as much body fat and you will have to re-adjust your nutrition and fitness training program to jump-start your metabolism.

Do not allow yourself to get off track by weighing yourself every day. Instead, focus your attention on energy levels, how you feel in your clothing and mental focus.

BODY MASS INDEX MEASUREMENTS

WHAT IS A BMI MEASUREMENT?

BMI stands for body mass index. BMI measurements are used in many health settings to help determine body fat in relation to one's height. As with any measurement, the BMI index is not an exact science.

There are many factors such as age, muscle mass and gender that are not considered in this measurement. Someone with an athletic body may register high on the BMI scale, but in all actuality have more lean mass than fat mass. Therefore, this measurement should be used with the existing knowledge that it isn't the most accurate measurement of body fat.

Although the BMI isn't an exact measure for body fat, it is a great tool to use if you want to determine whether you are at a healthy body weight for your height or at risk for certain health concerns. High BMI's (>30) have been linked to diseases such as hypertension, high cholesterol, diabetes and obesity. Finding your BMI is a simple process that does not require expensive tools or a trained professional.

HOW DO YOU CALCULATE YOUR BMI?

The only thing you need to calculate your BMI is a calculator and a piece of paper.

The first step in calculating your BMI is to know your current height and weight. If you do not know your current weight, find a scale and weigh yourself. If you are not aware of your height, find a measuring tape and have someone measure your height.

Follow the example below to determine your BMI by plugging in your height and weight. If you are not comfortable with numbers, you may search the World Wide Web to find a free BMI calculator to do the math for you.

Example: Amy is 150 pounds and 5 feet 8 inches (68 inches) tall. Try this one for practice and then plug in your measurements in order to calculate your own BMI.

BMI Equation: Weight (kg)/Height (m) squared

1. **Determine weight in kilograms.**

   Divide pounds by 2.2. (Dividing by 2.2 converts pounds into kilograms)

   (Ex). 150/2.2 = 68.2 kg

2. **Determine height in meters squared.**

   First, determine ht. in cm.

   (Ex). 68 inches x 2.54 = 172.72 cm.

   Next, divide ht. in cm. by 100 to get ht. in meters.

   (Ex). 172.72/100 = 1.73

   Then, square ht. in meters.

   (Ex). 1.73 x 1.73 = 2.98

3. **Divide weight in kg (68.2) by height in meters squared (2.98) = 23**

4. Go to the chart below and find whether or not Amy is at a healthy BMI. If your answer is yes, then you have calculated the right answer.

BMI CATEGORIES

BMI less than 18.5, falls within the "underweight" range.

BMI 18.5 to 24.9, it falls within the "normal" or "healthy weight" range.

BMI 25.0 to 29.9, it falls within the "overweight" range. Therefore, you may need to lose weight, especially if you have two or more of the risk factors for diseases associated with "overweight" range.

BMI 30.0 or higher falls within the "obese" range. Therefore, you should talk to your doctor or health care provider about weight loss options.

BMI >40, falls within the range of "morbid obesity" Therefore, you should talk to your doctor or health care provider about weight loss options and determine if you are healthy enough to exercise.

HOW FIT ARE YOU?

For many women, being fit means weighing a certain amount on the scale and wearing a particular clothing size. Although having a healthy weight is important for health reasons, it doesn't define whether or not someone is fit. Being fit is a combination of muscular strength, muscular endurance, flexibility and cardiovascular endurance.

Bye, bye scale, hello pushups!

The only tools needed to determine your current level of fitness is a stopwatch, partner and yoga mat.

Are you ready?

ONE-MINUTE SIT-UP TEST:

Purpose: This test is used to determine abdominal endurance and strength. Abdominal endurance and strength are important for core stability and back support.

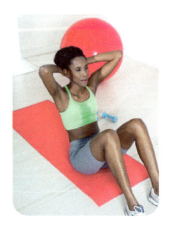

A. Lay on your back with knees bent. Fingers must be interlocked behind the neck and the back of hands must touch the mat. Another person holds your ankles with hands only. If you don't have someone to hold your ankles, place your feet under a firm and stable surface such as a couch.

B. On go, you or your partner will start the stop watch and you will bring your body up and bring your elbows to touch thighs. You will lower your body and return to the ground where only the upper portion of your back touches the ground. Repeat movement for one minute and then count the number of sit-ups completed. Record your numbers.

PUSH-UP TEST (UPPER BODY STRENGTH AND ENDURANCE):

Purpose: The one-minute push-up test is used to assess upper body strength and endurance.

A. Begin with body in push up position. A standard push up begins with the hands and toes touching the floor, the body and legs in a straight line, feet together, arms shoulder width apart with slight bend in elbows.

B. Keeping the back and knees straight, lower your body to a predetermined point, or until there is a 90-degree angle of the elbows, pause for a second and then return to the starting position with the arms extended without locking elbows. Repeat this action for one minute. Record your numbers.

C. If you do not have the upper body strength, perform push-ups on knees, this is considered the modified version.

3-MINUTE STEP-UP TEST

Purpose: The 3-Minute Step Test measures your aerobic (cardiovascular) fitness level based on how quickly your heart rate returns to normal after exercise.

A. Before test begins, measure your resting heart rate.

Measure your resting heart rate: To do this, turn your hand over so the palm of your hand is facing upwards towards the ceiling. Locate the top of your thumb and follow your thumb until you get to the ending point of your hand. From there, using your index and middle finger, locate your radial pulse (which is located inside the hand at the base of your thumb). Don't press too hard, but gently feel for a pulse. Once you have found a pulse, set your timer and count the number of times you feel a pulse for 15 seconds and then multiply this number by 4. This is your resting pulse rate. Record your numbers.

B. From there, locate a chair or bench that is at least 12 inches high. Stand in front of the bench or chair. Start the timer and slowly step on bench/chair with one foot. Then bring other foot on bench. Use a four-step cadence, "up-up-down-down" for 3 minutes with a steady pace. At any time you feel out of breath or tired, stop for a moment in a standing position. Stop immediately on completion of 3 minutes.

C. Take pulse immediately after 3 minutes as explained in step A. Multiply the number of beats you count by 4.

D. This number represents your heart rate after exercising.

Example: 22 beats X 4 = 88 beats per minute

The quicker your heart rate drops to its resting rate, means your cardiovascular system is becoming more conditioned. In 4-6 weeks you will re-do this test and your heart rate should not get as high and you should reach your resting heart rate quicker due to your heart being more conditioned. Remember this is a starting point; you're a work in progress.

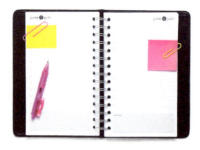

REASSESS, REASSESS, REASSESS

Once you gather your numbers and measurements, record them and place them in your fitness journal. Four to six weeks from your original assessment date, you will want to reassess your measurements and fitness testing. You will perform the exact tests you performed above, and then compare results.

If you have noticed a positive change in numbers (ex. more strength, better cardiovascular conditioning, decreased girth measurements, BMI and Heart Rate), your fitness-training program is working and it will be time to set new fitness goals.

If you're not improving, it is recommended to re-evaluate your fitness program and motivation. During your evaluation, be honest with yourself and hold yourself accountable. Identify areas that are hindering you from reaching your goals, and from there set a realistic plan of action to reach your desired destination.

If you have not reached your goal, don't result to negative self-talk, you are working on being the best version of yourself and negative self-talk won't get you there.

STEP 4. CREATE A PLAN OF ACTION

LET ME ASK you a question. Would you go on a road to trip to a particular destination without an address or directions?

WOULD YOU GO ON A ROAD TRIP WITHOUT A MAP OR DIRECTIONS?

More than likely your answer is no. The same principle applies for reaching your fitness goals. It is harder to reach your destination without direction. Therefore once you have your measurements and fitness assessment numbers recorded, it's time create a plan of attack to reach your desired fitness goals.

If your goal is to do more push-ups within a minute and build upper body strength, then a plan of action to build upper body strength is required. If you desire better cardiovascular conditioning, a cardiovascular program needs to be designed.

Whatever your goals, your plan of action needs to create the right steps to help you reach your destination.

How do you create a plan of action? Let's find out.

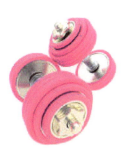

FIT JEWEL
Having no plan of action to get fit will leave you frustrated and distracted. Create a plan and work your plan, you're worth it!

CREATE YOUR PLAN OF ATTACK

THE FIRST STEP in creating your plan of action is to find physical activities and exercise that you enjoy. If you enjoy something, you are more likely to stick with it and reach your goals easier. Working out should be an exciting time to focus on yourself

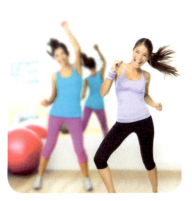

and not feel tortured during the process. Therefore, it is essential to find something you enjoy doing. Many gyms offer group fitness classes including kickboxing, Zumba, spin and boot camps. Try each one of these classes to determine which classes you enjoy most. Choose classes that are fun and are most beneficial to help you reach your fitness goal.

Fitness is about having fun. Move to your own beat. If you like to dance, just dance!

If you decide group fitness classes work for you, alternate classes to avoid overuse injuries and boredom. Overuse injuries are the result of performing the same movement patterns on a consistent basis. Constant movement patterns stress the same muscles and joints and can lead to chronic (long-term) or acute (short-term) injuries. In addition to possible overuse injuries, attending the same classes will eventually cause your body to hit a plateau and lead to limited changes in your body and cardiovascular conditioning levels.

DETERMINE HOW MANY DAYS TO EXERCISE

ONCE YOU DETERMINE which activities you enjoy, it's time to realistically determine how many days per week you are willing to dedicate to these activities. You know your commitments more than anyone else, therefore don't commit to more days than you can handle with your current lifestyle. If you can only do three days a week, some physical activity is better than no exercise at all. If you can't get all three days in, do what you can and don't fall into the "all or none" philosophy once you set your days of the week to exercise.

WHAT IS THE "ALL OR NONE" PHILOSOPHY?

THE "ALL OR none" philosophy is a belief that if you miss one session of your planned activity during the week than there is no point of going for the entire week. This is a negative philosophy and mentality that can keep you from reaching your fitness goal(s). Therefore, I will once again reiterate, be realistic about the amount of days you can commit to your fitness program and some exercise is better than no exercise.

KEEP MOVING - IT'S JUST LIFE!

IF WE LIVED in the perfect world, we could spend as much time as we wanted dedicated to getting fit, but unfortunately the world and our lives aren't perfect and we have to be flexible with getting enough physical activity in.

We get busy, emergencies and unexpected events happen, things come up that are out of our control and we sometimes get thrown off schedule, but when this happens, keep going and adapt.

FIVE TIPS TO KEEP YOUR BODY MOVING WHEN LIFE HAPPENS

1. If you can't make it to your normal scheduled class, try another class. If you normally go to a 6:00 pm class and you're running late, try a 6:30 pm class. If there isn't one available, get creative in the gym and try a new piece of cardio equipment or resistance training machine. Do not leave the gym without doing something healthy for yourself.

2. Can't make it to the gym? Go for a walk. You don't have to attend the gym to get fit. If you can't make it on a particular day, go for a walk. Walking is a great way to relieve stress and clear your mind.

3. Keep an extra set of gym clothes and shoes in your car. If you have to go back home to get your workout clothes, more than likely you're not going back to the gym. Therefore, always keep an extra set of gym clothes and shoes in your trunk. Consider this your emergency gym kit.

4. You wake up late - make the most of the time you have. If you don't wake up when the alarm goes off and all you have is 10 minutes to exercise, do something. Keep in mind doing 10 minutes of some exercise is better than no exercise at all.

5. Your boss tells you that you have to work later than planned. If you have to work longer than expected and you're going to miss your workout, take a brisk walk around your office building. If you have stair cases in your building, take the stairs for an allotted period of time. Don't panic, life happens, just keep moving.

STEP 5. DETERMINE YOUR MOTIVATION

WHAT'S YOUR MOTIVATION?

THE LAST STEP in beginning your fitness journey is to discover your motivation. Discovering your motivation may help you become more consistent with your fitness training program.

In order to discover how you are motivated, it's important to identify your motivation style.

ARE YOU INTRINSICALLY OR EXTRINSICALLY MOTIVATED?

Someone who is intrinsically motivated is self-motivated and reaches goals for self-gratification and not external rewards. Intrinsically motivated people are driven by something within themselves and do not need anyone to motivate them. They set goals for themselves and are motivated to accomplish those goals without any external reward or a required cheering squad.

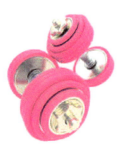

FIT JEWEL

What makes you want to move? Discover it and run with it!

Then there are those who are extrinsically motivated. Extrinsically motivated people are individuals who need an external force (such as rewards or praise from other people) to motivate them. They need consistent feedback and support to feel they are doing well and without support, they are less likely to complete the task they have started. Neither one of these motivational styles are wrong, we are individuals and are driven by different motivating factors.

If you are more geared towards being extrinsically motivated, below are a few tips for you.

TIPS FOR EXTRINSICALLY MOTIVATED PEOPLE

- Reward yourself with non-food related items when you met certain goals.
- Place a picture of what you want to look like on your fridge and in your training journal - this may help provide you with visual motivation.
- When you reach a goal, share it with someone in your support team. Sharing your success will help keep you motivated.

STEADY BUT GRADUAL PROGRESS

IF YOU'RE FEELING overwhelmed by all the steps you have just learned, exhale for a moment and tell yourself to focus on the process and not the outcome. Allow yourself the freedom to embrace this process without expectations of time. Your fitness journey is a jog and not a sprint, and I am confident that you will reach your destination if you give yourself time.

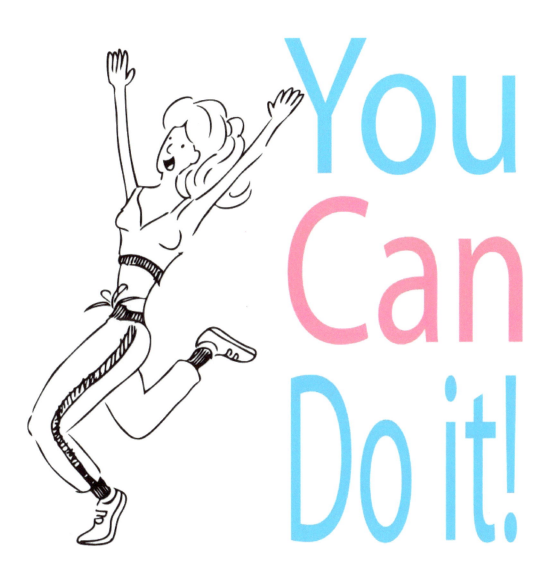

Can You Spot Reduce?

WE'RE MAKING GREAT PROGRESS AREN'T WE?

Let's do a recap! We've talked about how to identify your body type, how to set fitness goals based on your fitness assessments and much more up to this point. Now I want to talk about one of the most misleading beliefs for a woman trying to get into shape.

LET'S TALK ABOUT SPOT REDUCTION. YES, SPOT REDUCTION!

Unfortunately, millions of women believe that they can spot reduce or lose body fat in particular areas of their body by targeting a specific area by taking a pill or rubbing a gel on their trouble areas! Just think about all the commercials and advertisements that promise reduced cellulite (the appearance a fat cells that have escaped your connective tissue matrix) by taking a few pills or by just rubbing a topical gel on the skin.

We've all been hopeful that these products will work. I don't like to be the bearer of bad news, but here's the truth: you can't spot reduce. In fact, I will go even further and tell you that you can't change your fat into muscle.

Now that we have the truth out there, let's understand why.

YOUR CELLS NEVER COMPLETELY GO AWAY

Every woman was born with a certain amount of fat cells in her body and, as a result of increased caloric consumption, stress, hormonal changes and a lack of physical activity, her fat cells grow. When these stubborn fat cells grow, various physical changes occur that may be noticeable. A woman may no longer be able to fit into her clothing, and the numbers on the scale may go up.

WHY DOES THIS HAPPEN?

Unhealthy lifestyles such as poor dietary choices, smoking and limited physical activity leads to unused energy to be stored into our fat cells. When this occurs, your fat cells grow, resulting in weight gain and a fuller appearance in areas where you are more genetically prone to gain weight. For most women, this is the lower body and abdomen area. Applying a gel or taking a pill cannot shrink the fat cells in your buttocks or abdominal area alone.

Fat cells typically only shrink when we utilize the stored energy through exercise, increase our water intake to remove toxins that are known to store in fat, and eat a healthy amount of calories to decrease the body's surplus energy stores.

I know this may not be what you wanted to hear, but I want to be honest with you. The good news is you can change the appearance of cellulite on your body by increasing your lean muscle to body fat ratio. We will talk about this a little later.

Now let's talk about why you can't turn fat into muscle.

We've all heard the gimmicky commercials where spokespeople claim that a particular product helped them turn their fat into muscle. Allow me to explain, once and for all: Muscle cannot turn into fat, and fat cannot turn into muscle!

WHY NOT?

Muscle tissue and fat cells are two separate structures in the body. Muscle fibers are long active fibers that build and repair themselves when we lift weights. They come in two separate categories, fast twitch muscle fibers (tissues the body uses for explosive activities and exercises) and slow twitch muscle fibers (tissues the body uses for long distance activities such as running and lower intensity exercises. Muscle fibers are known to be highly metabolic and create more energy than fat cells.

Fat cells, on the other hand, are slow in metabolism, known to store toxins and can place you at risk for heart disease and other health issues when not maintained and controlled. Fat is a slow yellow tissue that is utilized at times during exercise depending on the intensity level of the exercise, but is generally lazy in nature.

All in all, these are two separate tissues and they do not convert! However, you can increase the size and strength of one (muscle tissue) and decrease the size of the other (fat) through exercise, so there is hope! Coupled together, cardiovascular activities, such as biking, walking, swimming or jogging, combined with lifting weights, can assist you in building lean toned muscle tissue that burns calories even at the state of rest.

Are you feeling more empowered with this knowledge?

Great, let's move on!

Why Won't Your Body Change?

Have you ever done endless hours of cardiovascular exercise, deceased your caloric intake through dieting, maybe even to lower-than-healthy levels, and yet your body stubbornly seems unwilling to change? Can you say frustrating! Has this ever happened to you? If it has, what you have experienced is known as adaptation. Yes, our bodies are amazing creations that have the ability to adapt to any external stress placed upon them.

WHAT DO I MEAN?

Allow me to paint a clearer image of adaptation. When we first begin exercising and our body isn't used to the particular activity we are performing the body is required to increase the amount of effort or energy required to perform that particular activity. As a result we experience increased heart rate and calorie burn allowing us to lose weight and make gains in our strength.

However after a certain period of time (adaptation period) the body requires less effort to perform the same task and you expend or exert less energy doing the same exercise as before. Let's use an example. When you first begin your weight lifting program you may only be able to perform 5 modified push-ups. Six weeks after you begin your program, you can complete 5-15 modified push-ups with minimal effort. What has occurred is what is known as neuromuscular adaptation. Your nerves and muscles have become coordinated and you have become stronger making your movements more fluid with less energy and coordination requirements.

SO, WHAT'S NEXT? I'M GLAD YOU ASKED.

In order to get even stronger and challenge your body on a new level you have to overload your body. Overload means you will have to increase the amount of weight, sets, repetitions and intensity of each one of your exercises. The body is very lazy and will only respond according to what you make it do. Yes, what you MAKE it do.

Therefore once you start your fitness training program and reach a point where you no longer see changes to your body, say to yourself "It's time to overload my body!"

OVERLOAD PROGRESSIVELY

When overloading your body be aware that this process must be a gradual process. In regards to increases in the amount of weight you lift, it is recommended that you go up in 2-5 pound increments and use the Rule of 2. The Rule of 2 states that if you can perform 2 more repetitions at the end of your set, then it is time to add more weight. When adding more weight, ensure at all times to keep proper posture.

 In the areas of cardiovascular activities try adding 5-10 minute increments and increase your intensity while performing these activities on a bi-weekly or monthly basis. It is also advisable to perform your cardiovascular activities on different machines in order to avoid overuse or movement pattern injuries.

Having this information will allow you to have a better understanding of what really happens inside of your body and what's required to make the necessary changes in order to see your body continually make changes.

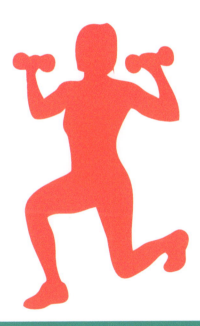

INCREASE YOUR REPS, INCREASE YOUR SETS, INCREASE YOUR INTENSITY!

PART 2

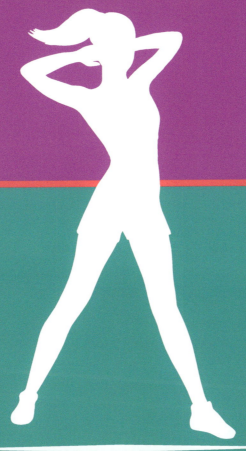

YOU KNOW IT GIRL!

Before You Begin

Before you make the decision to pick up a dumbbell or workout on a weight machine, it is important to understand a few key lifting techniques and training methods. These techniques and training methods will help you avoid injury and provide you with information to navigate through the Iron Palace (gym) with more confidence.

LIFTING TECHNIQUES

WHENEVER YOU PERFORM an exercise (either on a machine or with free weights), there are two primary phases of movements. These phases of movement include an eccentric and concentric phase.

The concentric phase of a movement occurs when the muscle contracts or shortens. If you were executing a bicep curl, curling the weight up is the concentric phase of the movement.

The opposite, or opposing movement, is called the eccentric movement. The eccentric phase of movement involves lengthening or releasing the weight back to the starting position. If you were performing a dumbbell bicep curl and released your hand and allow the dumbbell to move downward away from your body, this would be the eccentric phase.

Each phase of movement challenges the muscles from a different level of difficulty, and one cannot be completed without the other. Therefore, it is important to only lift an amount of weight you can control during each phase of the movement. Never jeopardize form to lift heavier weight.

If an amount of weight is too heavy, choose a lighter weight. Once again I will reiterate, do not sacrifice form to lift a heavier amount of weight. Choosing to lift heavy weight in which you can't lift properly through both phases of movement can result in acute and permanent injuries.

LIFTING POSTURE STANDING

WHILE PERFORMING ANY lifting movement in a standing position, feet are to be positioned slightly apart with knees slightly bent. Core or abdominals are held in tight, with shoulder blades back and chest up. Never round your back and be aware of your posture at all times.

POSTURE ON MACHINES

EACH MACHINE IS created to operate in a fixed range of motion meaning you can only move the machine in a predetermined movement pattern. This is beneficial in many ways, but proper posture is still required while using machines. Proper posture involves controlled movements and keeping core engaged at all times throughout the exercise.

PROPER BREATHING

PROPER BREATHING CONSISTS of inhaling at the starting phase of the movement, before the beginning of the lift (concentric phase), and exhaling during the release of the weight (eccentric phase). Holding your breath while lifting can cause dizziness and create a lack of oxygen to working muscles.

TRAINING METHODS

WE HAVE DISCOVERED proper lifting techniques, now it's time to learn different resistance training methods. The following resistance training methods are the most common and most applicable.

SPLIT TRAINING

SPLIT TRAINING IS a term used to identify how each muscle group is divided and trained. Using the split training method ensures each muscle group is trained on a consistent basis, to avoid muscular imbalances and muscular injuries from under and overdeveloped muscles.

HOW DO YOU CREATE A SPLIT TRAINING ROUTINE THAT IS RIGHT FOR YOU?

TO CREATE YOUR individualized split, determine how many days a week you can dedicate to resistance training. Once you have completed this task, decide which muscle groups you want to train together or by themselves (ex. Biceps and Triceps, Back and Chest). Some research suggests training your muscles in a push/pull fashion, but you make the decision. This method is believed to create muscular balances if done properly.

Training in a push/pull fashion involves training muscles that allow you to perform pushing and pulling movements within the same training session. Doing a push-up is considered a pushing movement (which uses your chest muscles), followed by seated dumbbells rows (which is a pulling movement) which work the back muscles.

Split training is designed based on individual preference, and your split may not mirror your girlfriends. Once you create your split schedule, it does not have to be set in stone. Changing the muscle groups and the days, you train them are beneficial both mentally and physically.

Possible Disadvantage of the Split Training Method

Although split training is a great training method, it is important to consider your current level of fitness before you create your split training routine.

Spilt training typically focuses on training one or two body parts per training session. Typically, the volume or the number of sets and repetitions you perform using this training method places more stress on your muscles. Placing a great amount of stress on untrained muscles can lead to excessive soreness and injuries. Therefore, if you are not at a training level where you can perform split training, full body training may be more advantageous for you.

ADVANTAGES OF SPLIT TRAINING

A BENEFIT OF split training for seasoned lifters is the ability to train a weak muscle group(s). With this method of training, you can focus on that particular group during your training session and perform more sets which can assist in strengthening your weaker muscle groups.

EXAMPLE OF SPLIT TRAINING

Monday:	**Biceps/Triceps/Abs**
Tuesday:	**Chest/Back**
Wednesday:	**Off**
Thursday:	**Shoulders/Abs**
Friday:	**Legs/Abs**
Saturday:	**Off**

FULL BODY TRAINING

AS THE NAME states, full body training is a method that targets each major muscle group within one training session. Full body training is a great method for beginners and for individuals who do not have enough time to devote to a split training regimen.

Full body training targets each muscle group, but it doesn't stress each individual muscle group as efficiently as split training. When you are doing a full body training session, you are typically performing one or two exercises per muscle group. This will help you tone, but to experience continual muscle growth, you will eventually need to stress each muscle group beyond full body training.

EXAMPLE OF FULL BODY TRAINING

2 sets per exercise, 12 to 15 repetitions

	Set 1	Set 2
Legs	**Lunges**	**Squats**
Biceps	**Bicep Curls**	**Hammer Curls**
Triceps	**Triceps Extensions**	**Triceps Kickbacks**
Shoulders	**Lateral Shoulder Raises**	**Front Shoulder Raises**
Back	**One-arm Rows**	**Seated Rows**
Abs	**Crunches**	**Leg Lifts**

SUPER SETTING

SUPER SETTING REQUIRES performing one exercise for a primary muscle group, followed immediately by performing an exercise for its opposing muscle group. Super setting keeps your muscles in balance due to the consistency of training both sides of your muscle group.

Super setting will cut back on gym time and allow the body to maintain balance within each muscle group.

EXAMPLE OF SUPER SETTING

Biceps/Triceps (bicep curls followed immediately by triceps extensions)

Back/Chest (lat pull downs, followed immediately by pushups)

Quads/Hamstrings (leg extensions, followed immediately by hamstring curls)

GIANT SET

PERFORMING A GIANT set requires choosing a particular muscle group and choosing four to five different exercises for that particular group.

After choosing your exercises, perform each exercise in a circuit fashion, moving from one exercise to another without rest until the set is complete.

Create your giant set based on your current fitness level. You can begin with two to three different exercises, and then progressively increase the amount of exercises as you become stronger and better conditioned.

EXAMPLE OF A GIANT SET

Muscle Group: Shoulders

Lateral shoulder raises	10 repetitions
Front shoulder raises	10 repetitions
Seated shoulder press	10 repetitions
Rear deltoid raises	10 repetitions

CIRCUIT TRAINING

CIRCUIT TRAINING INVOLVES performing a group of exercises in a continuous fashion, and not reaching a stopping point until each exercise is completed.

Circuit training is believed to be an effective training method for people who are short on time and desire more cardiovascular conditioning.

Cardiovascular conditioning is a result of a continually elevated heart rate throughout the circuit.

EXAMPLE OF CIRCUIT TRAINING

Remember to perform each exercise in a continual fashion before you reach a state of rest.

Stationary lunges	12 repetitions
Standing bicep curls	12 repetitions
Triceps kickbacks	12 repetitions
Standing shoulder press	12 repetitions
Modified pushups	8-10 repetitions
Crunches	12 repetitions

INTERVAL TRAINING

INTERVAL TRAINING INVOLVES performing short periods of high-intensity exercise followed immediately by the same activity at a lower intensity.

Studies show interval training burns more calories than regular steady state (performing exercise at the same pace over a period of time) physical activities.

Intervals can be created during any activity.

EXAMPLE OF INTERVAL TRAINING

An example of interval training would be sprinting on the treadmill at a 6.9 speed for 30 seconds followed by jogging at a speed of 4.0 for one minute. Repeat interval five times)

DETERMINE YOUR SETS, REPETITIONS, AND WEIGHT

ONE OF THE most common questions women have when it comes to resistance training is, "How much weight should I lift ito reach my goals?"

The amount of weight you lift is based on your fitness goals. If you desire to build toned, lean muscles, you will perform exercises with light weight five to 15 pounds) within a repetition range of 15 to 20 repetitions while performing at least three sets of each exercise.

If your goal is to build an athletic body with more dense muscle tissue, you will lift heavier weight (15 pounds or more) within a range of eight to 15 repetitions performing at least 4-5 sets of each exercise.

As a rule of thumb, the heavier weight you use, the fewer repetitions you will perform. This builds strength and muscle density.

The lighter weight you use, the higher repetitions you will perform. This will create lean, toned muscles.

WAIT I STILL HAVE QUESTIONS!

WALKING INTO A room full of men with bulging biceps can leave you doubting the choice you have made to start a resistance training program, but equipping yourself with the proper armor before you enter the Iron Palace will give you more confidence and the ability to freely navigate your way through.

Entering the Iron Palace may seem intimidating right now, but below you will discover answers to the most frequently asked questions from women regarding resistance and cardiovascular training. Knowing the answers to these questions may help you feel more confident when you enter the Iron Palace.

FAQS REGARDING RESISTANCE AND CARDIOVASCULAR TRAINING

Q.

HOW MANY DAYS A WEEK SHOULD I LIFT?

A.

It is recommended that beginners start with two to three days per week performing total body workouts or using machines. The beginning of your fitness training program should be gradual, with an emphasis on technique or lifting form. Training too frequently or intensely at this stage of your fitness-training program could lead to injuries and early burn out.

Intermediate and advanced trainees can train four to five days per week, allowing at least 48 hours of rest per muscle group. If you are in a training rut, revamp your entire fitness training program by overloading your body with more repetitions, heavier weight, different exercises, and less rest time in between sets.

A rule of thumb - if you have been using the same fitness training program for more than six weeks, it is time to update your program.

Q.

MACHINES OR FREE WEIGHTS?

A.

Both. Using a combination of machines and free weights can assist you in reaching your fitness goals.

MACHINES

Machines are great for beginners, they are easy to operate and provide step-by-step instructions. Most machines provide pictorials to identify which muscle groups are used during the execution of the movement. Machines are created to move in a fixed range of motion that prevents improper form and this is beneficial to individuals who aren't experienced with resistance training. Using machines does not require a high level of coordination, balance or strength for beginners.

FREE WEIGHTS

Using free weights requires proper knowledge of form in order to execute each desired exercise. Using free weights also requires balance, coordination and core strength. Free weights engage more muscular activity than using machines and can challenge the body in a different manner than machines. More muscle engagement means more calories burned. More calories burned means a more lean and toned body.

Q.

HOW MUCH WEIGHT SHOULD I LIFT?

A.

BEGINNERS

Beginners are recommended to find an amount of weight that will allow them to perform 12 to 15 repetitions safely throughout an entire range of movement. When reaching the 15th repetition if the weight is still challenging to lift, stay with that amount of weight. Once you reach a point where the weight is no longer challenging, make small increases in weight. You can progress from 5 lbs. to 8 lbs. then to 10 lbs. This process is known as progressive resistance training.

INTERMEDIATE AND ADVANCED TRAINEES

Select an amount of weight heavy enough that will allow you to execute eight to 15 repetitions with proper form. If you reach your 15th repetition and the weight is not challenging, increase the weight by 5 lbs.

Q.

HOW MANY REPETITIONS DO I PERFORM?

A.

The number of repetitions performed for any exercise is determined by your fitness goals.

For Power Moves

- 2 to 3 repetitions
- Heavy weight
- This will help athletes develop power and explosiveness.

For Muscular Strength

- 8 to 15 repetitions

- Moderate to heavy weight

- This will help build lean and dense muscle tissue.

For Muscular Endurance

- 15 to 20 repetitions

- Light weight

- This will help tone lean muscles.

Q.

HOW MUCH CARDIO SHOULD I DO?

A.

Cardiovascular activity should be a part of every person's fitness training program.

According to The American College of Sports Medicine and the American Heart Association, perform at least 60 minutes of moderate to vigorous physical activity most days of the week.

However, the specific amount of cardio you need varies from person to person and depends on the following factors:

- Daily caloric intake

- Exercise intensity and frequency

- Your metabolic rate (rate of substance breakdown)

- Your current fitness level (sedentary individuals will require a gradual increase in cardiovascular activities)

- Your body fat percentage

- Your current weight

- Your fitness goals

BEGINNERS

Perform at least 25 to 30 minutes of light-to-moderate intensity cardiovascular activities most days of the week. Gradually progress where you can perform 35 to 45 minutes of continuous cardiovascular activities as your heart and lungs become more conditioned.

INTERMEDIATE AND ADVANCED

Perform at least 40 minutes to one hour, including intervals.

Q.

WHAT IS A HEART RATE?

A.

Heart rate is the number of beats the heart takes within one minute. There is a direct correlation between heart rate and workload (work performed). As workload or intensity increases, heart rate will increase. To keep track of your heart rate, you may purchase a heart rate monitor. Wearing a heart rate monitor will help gauge your intensity levels at all times.

Q.

HOW DO I FIND MY PULSE RATE TO DETERMINE HOW INTENSE I AM EXERCISING?

A.

You can determine your pulse rate by using your radial pulse (arm).

In order to locate your radial pulse, turn your hand over with thumb turned in an outward position. Start at tip of thumb and go all the way to the base of your thumb and move about half an inch from base of thumb using index and middle fingers and search for a pulse.

Once pulse is located, count the number of heart beats for 10 seconds. Multiply this number by six. This number will give you your heart rate.

Setting a target heart rate will give you an intensity level to reach for while exercising.

Q.

IN WHAT ORDER SHOULD I PERFORM MY EXERCISES?

A.

If you are training to become powerful, power moves are performed first in your workout program. Power moves require lifting heavy amounts of weight that fatigue your neuromuscular system and should not be performed when you are fatigued. power moves should occur at the beginning of your fitness routine (ex. Plyometrics)

Next, you will want to perform exercises that require the use of larger muscles (legs, chest, back) or multi-joint exercises. These exercises require more energy to perform, therefore, should be done before performing single-joint exercises which require less effort.

Last to be performed are smaller or single-joint exercises (shoulders, triceps, biceps). To avoid fatigue, do not train smaller muscles first. Training your smaller muscle groups first will cause you to fatigue quicker and lead to a less-than-optimal training session for your larger muscle groups.

Q.

HOW MUCH REST TIME SHOULD I TAKE IN BETWEEN SETS?

A.

The amount of rest time taken in between sets is determined by the amount of weight used and the intensity level at which you perform the exercise. Performing powerful and explosive movements may require 3-5 minutes of rest. This amount of rest time is needed to produce more energy and allows your neurological system time to recuperate.

For lower intensity exercises, rest for 30-90 seconds and no longer.

Q.

HOW MUCH REST TIME SHOULD I TAKE OFF BETWEEN WORKOUT SESSIONS?

A.

Resistance training involves breaking down muscle fibers (muscle tissue) that result in muscular soreness referred to as D.O.M.S. (Delayed Onset Muscle Soreness). The body naturally repairs these micro tears during rest. Therefore, not getting the proper amount of rest can lead to overtraining, diminishes in strength and a weakened immune system and fatigue.

Therefore, it is recommended to allow at least 48 hours of rest time between the training of each muscle group. If you are afraid to take a complete day off, you may take part in activities called active rest. During active rest, you are performing more leisure-based activities such as walking the dog, gardening or maybe going for a casual walk.

Below are signs of training burnout and overtraining. Familiarize yourself with these signs and be mindful that more isn't always better!

Signs of Burnout or Overtraining

- Weakened immune system (more susceptible to infections)
- Decrease in motivation
- Excessive muscle soreness
- Irritability
- Decreases in strength
- Easily distracted

Q.

CAN MUSCLE TURN INTO FAT?

A.

No, muscle and fat are two separate types of tissue. One cannot convert into the other.

When muscle tissue is not stressed by lifting adequate amounts of weight (resistance), the muscles atrophy (become smaller).

When a person gains fat weight, it is not a result of muscle tissue turning into fat; it is a result of an increase in size of their fat cells.

Q.

SHOULD I DO CARDIO OR WEIGHTS?

A.

To create a strong, lean and toned physique you need to incorporate both.

To all of my resistance training enthusiasts, resistance training is great for building lean muscle tissue, but without cardiovascular activity, that six pack you have been working so hard to create may not be seen. Body fat can threaten to hide your hard-earned muscle and one of the ways you can show off what you have worked hard for is to incorporate cardiovascular activities into your regular fitness training sessions along with clean eating.

To my cardio queens, if the only thing you do is cardio, I want to encourage you to step into the Iron Palace and begin a resistance training program. Cardiovascular activities will change your size, but it will not change the shape of your body. Resistance training will help build a toned, calorie-burning machine. Muscle tissue is a dense, active tissue that burns calories even at the state of rest.

Learn the Lingo

Below you will learn many of the terminologies or lingos used in the gym world. Familiarize yourself with this terminology and you will become even more comfortable when you step into the Iron Palace!

Principle of Individual Differences - Everyone has a different genetic makeup and different training needs. Your fitness training program needs to be designed around your individuality. Your friend's training program may not work for you.

Principle of Adaptation - The body is a dynamic creation that changes when constant external (resistance training/weights) forces are applied. In order for your body to grow, continue to challenge your body with more repetitions, sets and volume of training.

Principle of Specificity - The only way to master a particular exercise or skill is to execute that particular exercise or skill on a regular basis. Specificity training is a very big principle in the athletic world. In order for a swimmer to become better at swimming, he/she has to swim. If you want to become great at a particular exercise, perform that exercise on a regular basis and your body will eventually adapt.

Principle of Progression - Placing too much stress or load on your body in a short period of time can lead to injuries. Therefore, gradually increase the amount of weight and intensity of each exercise you perform. Doing this will prevent excessive soreness, over training and mental burnout.

Principle of Use/Disuse - It is a cliché, but it is true. "If you don't use it, you lose it." When muscles are under consistent tension or stress, they adapt and grow. This process is called hypertrophy.

When muscles are not stressed, they become smaller and weaker. A process called atrophy. If you incorporate a resistance training program for a period of time, then stop for a longer period of time, your muscles will atrophy (become smaller). No stress means no growth.

Principle of Overload - Once the body adapts to a stress or load, it has to be challenged with more stress or load. Continuing to perform the same exercises, sets, repetitions and rest time does not challenge the body enough to force it to change. You have to overload your body and there is no way around this principle.

Abduction - movement away from the midline of the body (e.g. doing seated abductions on a machine). In this exercise, you bring your legs from an inward position to an outward position.

Adduction – movement towards the midline of the body e.g. doing seated adductions on a machine). In this exercise, you bring your legs from an outward position to an inward position.

Atrophy - loss of muscle due to lack of training stimulus.

Cardiovascular - pertains to your heart, veins and arteries.

Concentric - upward or contraction phase of a movement/muscle shortens (muscle contracts).

Dorsi Flexion - pointing toes upward towards the ceiling.

Eccentric - downward or negative phase of a movement/muscle lengthens (muscle relaxes).

Elbow extension - movement resulting in an increase of the elbow joint (triceps extension) of the body. These planes of motion allow the body to move in a certain direction and help identify movements of particular joints.

Elbow flexion - movement resulting in a decrease of the elbow joint (performing a bicep curl).

Extension - increases the angle of a joint (performing leg extensions is an example of knee extension).

Flexibility - range of motion around a joint.

Flexion - decreases the angle of a joint (oerforming a bicep curls is an example of elbow flexion).

Hyperextend - to go beyond a point or distance.

Hypertrophy - muscular growth due to training stimulus.

Lateral - side movement (e.g. lateral shoulder raises).

Muscular Endurance - the ability to continually exert force against a resistance.

Maximum heart rate - the highest number of times your heart beats in one minute.

Muscular Strength - the ability to exert a maximal amount of force against resistance.

Plantar Flexion - pointing toes downward.

Primary muscle - intended targeted muscle you want to train (when performing bicep curls, primary muscle is the bicep).

Respiratory - pertains to your lungs.

Repetition - repeated movement of a particular exercise.

Rotation - side-to-side or left-to-right movement of the trunk (top part of body) (e.g. performing Russian Twists) or neck.

Set - designated amount of repetitions.

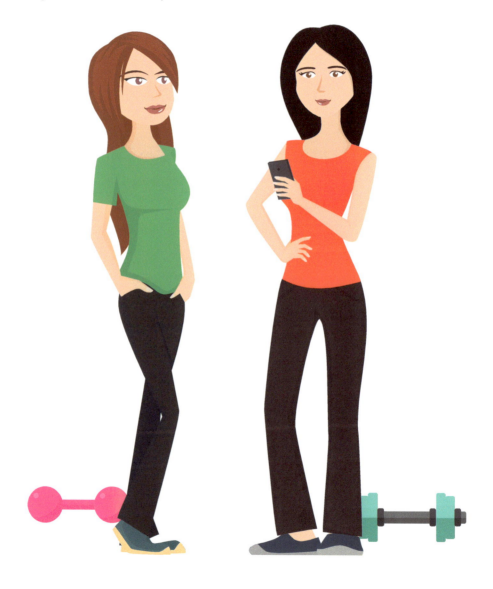

DON'T SPEND ALL OF YOUR GYM TIME TALKING!

SOCIAL HOUR IS OVER!

THIS ISN'T CLUB TALK

Being around like-minded fitness enthusiasts at the gym can help you reach your fitness goals and possibly lead you to making lifetime friendships. However, working out at the gym can also be a place where you can get distracted from reaching your goals.

DISTRACTED, WHO ME?

As women, many of us have one thing in common, we love to socialize. Yes, many of us are social butterflies, and this can be a great thing at the right time and right place, but it is not social hour when you walk through the gym doors. You are there to train and focus on your fitness goals.

Does this mean that you have to be unfriendly and non-sociable? Not at all, but it does mean that 90 percent of your time shouldn't be spent talking. Talking and not working out will prevent you from reaching your fitness goals. If you enjoy chatting, have your talks during your cool down and stretching.

Before we continue, let me share a pet peeve of mine.

If you are new to the gym, you may not be able to relate to this, but if you're a "gy-mette," you will know exactly what I mean. Let me paint the picture for you.

PLEASE DON'T DISTRACT ME!

It has been a long day at work and all you can think about is getting to the gym and having a grueling workout. OK, maybe you don't enjoy the grueling aspect of training, but follow me anyway. You rush to the gym and can't wait for some alone time.

You change into your training gear and are ready to train. You walk out into the Iron Palace and you begin your warm up. You have your music on the right song and you are starting to feel your body's core temperature increase. Ten minutes of a general warm up and you are ready to attack the IRON.

You get your gloves on and all you can think about is the feeling of iron held in your hands. You scope out your weapon of mass destruction and head in that direction. On the way there you have the eye of the tiger and all of a sudden someone stops and says "Hi, how are you?" You do not want to lose your focus and at the same time, you don't want to be rude. You say, "I'm great thanks." Another question comes. "So how is work?" You think, "Oh no, if I do not walk away more questions are going to follow."

Sure enough, you try to walk off and the person keeps talking. You are cooling down and someone has taken the equipment you wanted to use. Can you say frustrated? If you are laughing right about now, you know exactly what I am talking about.

The gym is a great place to meet people, but keep in mind - it isn't social hour when you are there. It's great to talk, but make your conversations polite and brief. Don't spend the majority of your time talking with friends or associates. If you do, you are losing time that could be invested in you transforming your body. How can you build a fit body if you spend the majority of your time talking?

A rule of thumb to keep in mind is - time spent in the gym does not automatically mean time spent on training. I frequently meet women who share that their fitness program just isn't working. When I ask them if they are in the gym for social hour or to train, many of the responses correspond with the latter.

If you are talking more than you're working, more than likely your mind is not focused on exercising. Therefore, here's your new mantra - "When it's time to train, it's time to train." Save the talking for cardio time.

AVOID WASTING GYM TIME

Talk during rest time: It is great having friends at the gym, but keep in mind you are there to train and not have social hour. Talk during your rest time between sets, but stay focused on why you're there.

Plan ahead of time: Have a plan of action before you hit the gym. Know which muscle(s) you are going to train and what exercises you are going to do before you arrive. Having a plan of attack will keep you from wondering around not sure of what to do.

Don't wait around: If a machine you want is occupied, politely ask the individual when they are going to be finished. Do not waste time waiting for a particular machine. Do another exercise and come back at a later time.

Perform exercises in a circuit fashion: A circuit involves choosing at least four different exercises for the entire body, and performing one exercise then immediately performing another without reaching a state of rest until all exercises are complete. Training in this fashion will keep your heart rate up and decrease gym time.

Double check your gym bag: Before leaving home, double check your gym bag to make sure you have socks, gym shoes, training clothes and hair ties. This will help you from having to go back home or stop at the store to purchase these items. This saves time and money.

Bring your own water: Have enough water to avoid frequent trips to the water fountain. Carry a large container to hold water instead of little 16 oz bottles that require many refills.

Fuel up: Eat a source of protein and complex carbohydrate at least one hour before your workout. Not having enough fuel can hinder your workout and prevent you from fully exerting yourself.

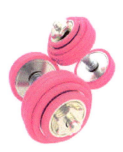

FIT JEWEL

Talk during your rest time between sets, but stay focused on why you're there.

FIT GIRL'S GYM ETIQUETTE

GYM ETIQUETTE 101

IF YOU ARE newcomer to the gym enviornent, this class will be new to you, however, if you're a seasoned veteran, this will be a refresher course.

KNOW THE RULES!

After spending many years in the gym, you become aware of what is acceptable and what is not. There are spoken and unspoken rules at the gym and now that you are going to be a part of this culture, it is important that you learn proper gym etiquette. The rules are as follows:

RULE 1: DON'T SIT IN SAUNA WITHOUT CLOTHES

We are all women, but there is something very awkward about having someone in the nude right in front of you doing things that most people would consider private. Being comfortable in your own skin is great, but be aware that there are other people who may not feel comfortable with you walking around in the nude. Embrace your body, but please put a towel on.

RULE 2: DON'T USE BATHROOM STALLS TO CHANGE CLOTHES

The bathroom should be used just for what is has been created for. If you are un-comfortable changing in front of other people it's understandable, but please don't change in the bathroom. Doing this holds the line up when other people need to use the restroom. Please be considerate and go into the shower area or other private designated area and change. Normally there is more space in these areas, and you will not hold up the restrooms.

RULE 3: NO PERFUME OVERLOAD

There is a time and place for everything, but wearing heavy amounts of perfume to the gym is definitely not the right time or place. Instead of using heavy perfumes that may affect other people, try a light body spray.

RULE 4: NO MACHINE HOARDING

Depending on the time of day, the gym can become overly crowded. If this is the case, you may have to share equipment with other people. If this happens, be open and willing to share. If you are working on a machine and taking a rest, allow someone else to use the machine during your rest time. Be friendly and respectful to everyone and if you are not using a machine, do not sit and talk on the machine. This hinders other people from using the machine.

RULE 5: DO NOT INTERRUPT

It is an unspoken rule, but a very important one. Do not interrupt someone during a set. If someone is in the middle of lifting weights or performing an exercise, wait until they are done before you interrupt them. It is rude and can break someone's focus if you speak to them while they are executing a movement. If you need to ask a question, wait until that person has completed with their set. If they are not finished, do not stand and wait. Walk away and come back when they are finished.

RULE 6: NO CELL PHONE ON GYM FLOOR

Cell phones can be a huge distraction to you and others. Talking on the phone while working out can be dangerous and annoying to others around you. If you need to talk, find a quiet place in the gym to excuse yourself. Some gyms do not allow members to talk on cell phones. If you train at a gym that has this rule, respect this rule and set an example to others.

If you are allowed to use your cell phone, keep in mind that other people come to the gym to de-stress and loud conversations on your cell phone can be disturbing.

RULE 7: MAKE A MESS, CLEAN YOUR MESS

It is unhealthy and very inconsiderate to leave your sweat on machines, mats or other equipment. Hundreds of people train at the gym and leave behind bacteria and certain viruses on a daily basis. Therefore, in order to help prevent the spread of germs and avoid getting sick, wipe down your equipment after each use. If there isn't any cleaner available, don't be afraid to ask gym staff to provide you with some antibacterial cleaner.

PREVENT THE SPREAD OF HARMFUL BACTERIA

- Wash hands before and after using restroom.

- Wipe machines off prior to use and immediately afterwards.

- If you are sick, stay at home.

- If you sneeze, do so towards the inside of your elbow. This will keep you from using your hands and then touching equipment.

- If you perspire heavily, bring a towel in order to keep your surrounding area clean.

- If your gym is out of sanitizer, nicely request to have the bottles refilled and spray equipment after every use.

- If you are using a mat to exercise, please be polite and clean it and then put it back when you are done. No one wants to search for a mat or lie on a mat that is covered in sweat.

- Cover any open cuts or wounds. Bacteria can get into open areas and cause infection.

- Do not place hands around your eyes or mouth during your workout.

- Wash hands prior to leaving the gym. Although the gym is a place to get fit and healthy, there's a lot of unwanted bacteria lurking around.

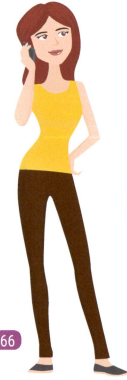

Talking on your cell phone while others are working out can be distracting to them and it can also hinder you from effectively focusing on your workout. Allow this time to be only for emergency calls. Besides, this is time dedicated for yourself, why let others interrupt you?

PART 3

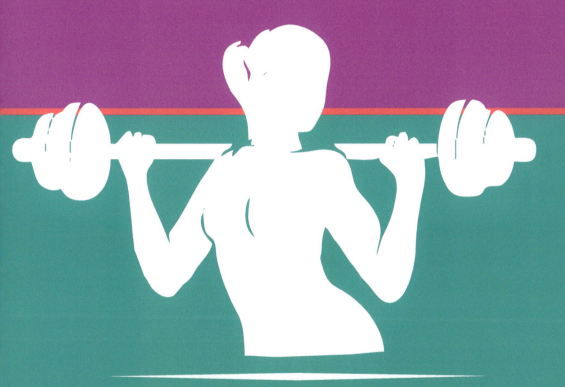

YES WOMEN LIFT!

Cardio Fit

ARE YOU THE QUEEN OF CARDIO?

DO YOU OFTEN find yourself doing hour-long cardio sessions with the hope of losing weight?

For many women, performing endless hours of cardio has become the solution to weight loss and getting into shape.

Although cardio can assist you in losing weight, doing endless hours of cardio will not ultimately get your body into the best shape compared to lifting weights.

You may have been taught that this is the only way to reach your fitness and weight loss goals, but I would like to share a better way to help you reap more benefits from doing less cardio.

HOW DOES THAT SOUND?

DO LESS AND REAP MORE

ALTHOUGH STEADY STATE (exercising at same intensity level for a period of time) cardio has its benefits, interval training can be more beneficial and require less time.

Studies have shown that performing 15-20 minutes of interval training can burn more calories than performing 40-45 minutes of steady state cardio if done at the appropriate intensity level. Therefore, why spend endless hours doing steady state cardio, when you can spend less time and gain more results by doing interval training?

INTERVAL WHAT?

WHAT IS INTERVAL TRAINING?

Interval training consists of performing short bursts of high intensity activity followed by short periods of lower intensity activity. You can create an interval on any piece of cardio equipment, with running or walking.

An example of a jog/sprint interval could consist of sprinting to a certain landmark (such as a mail box) and then jogging to another land mark (such as a stop sign).

The intensity of your high bursts is based on your current level of fitness and as with any physical activity, interval training should be done in moderation and safely. Interval training requires higher bursts of movements, and if done too fast for beginners could result in injuries.

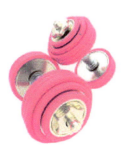

FIT JEWEL
Doing endless hours of cardio will not ultimately get your body into the best shape.

Therefore, it is recommended beginners perform intervals 1-2 times per week in the beginning of your fitness program and increase the frequency as your cardiovascular condition improves.

For individuals who are intermediate or advanced, perform intervals 3-4 days per week allowing yourself at least 48 hours of rest per week. Too much of any good thing is bad for you.

HOW DO YOU CREATE AN INTERVAL?

DETERMINE YOUR CURRENT fitness level and cardiovascular conditioning (beginner, intermediate or advanced).

Determine how much cardio you desire to perform.

Choose a machine(s), or decide if you want to perform walking or running intervals.

Based on your fitness level, create an interval for a desired amount of time.

The amount of time you rest is based on the intensity of activity (e.g., you can sprint on the treadmill for 20 seconds and then walk for 30 seconds).

The higher the intensity of each activity, typically the longer the rest/recovery time (e.g., If you sprint for 30 seconds you may need 45 seconds to 1 minute to recover by jogging or walking at a slower pace).

Interval Tip: Most cardio machines have programmed intervals. If you are not sure how to use your gym equipment, do not be afraid to ask for assistance.

INTENSITY PLEASE!

IN ORDER TO get the most bang for your buck, make sure you are putting in the right amount of INTENSITY into your intervals.

Intensity is the amount of effort you put into your exercise and one way to determine your effort is to use the R.P.E. (Rate of Perceived Exertion) scale.

WHAT IS THE R.P.E. SCALE?

The R.P.E. is a subjective scale using the numbers zero through ten to rank your intensity (effort put into activity) during your physical activity.

By learning this scale, you can determine if you are putting enough effort into your interval sessions. This scale can be used for your resistance training routine as well.

R.P.E. SCALE	
0	NOTHING AT ALL
1	VERY LIGHT
2	FAIRLY LIGHT
3	MODERATE
4	SOMEWHAT HARD
5	HARD
6	
7	VERY HARD
8	
9	
10	VERY HARD (MAXIMAL Intensity)

ARE YOU TIRED OF THE SAME OLD THING?

DOING CARDIO ON a treadmill or elliptical can eventually become boring and cause overuse injuries due to performing the same movement patterns on a regular basis.

Besides, don't you get tired of the same old thing? Then, why not get creative with your cardio?

It's time to think outside the box and try the following cardio blast program.

This cardio blast routine will challenge your body by giving your mind a break from the monotony of your daily grind on the treadmill.

Items needed: Jump rope, bench or stable chair and medicine ball

Step 1: Gather needed items: Jump rope, bench or stable chair, medicine ball, your body.

Step 2: Identify your skill level (beginner, intermediate or advanced) and follow recommended sets and repetitions.

Step 3: Perform each exercise. At any point, adjust sets and repetitions according to your skill level and personal difficulty.

The following exercises are performed in a circuit fashion. Perform one exercise then move immediately to the next exercise without resting. Complete each exercise and then come to a state of rest.

General Warm-Up: Perform 5-10 minutes of light activity, such as jogging in place or walking on treadmill.

Jump Rope: Body standing straight with slight bend in knees. Hold rope lightly in hands. Turn rope, maintain soft bend in knees, stay on the base of feet. Do not pound feet on ground.

Step Ups: Stand in front of chair or bench with feet slightly apart and bend in knees. Keep upper body straight with core tight, arms by side. Slowly step up on bench with left foot, then right foot. Step back with opposite foot, until both feet are on ground, then repeat.

Med Ball Throw Downs: While standing straight, position med ball chest level using both hands. With a slight bend in knees, move body in an upward movement, bringing ball over head and then throwing ball toward ground. Let ball rebound, then catch. Repeat movement.

Line Hops: Create an imaginary line on the surface you are using. Stand behind imaginary line. While standing straight with slight bend in knees, jump forward over line, then jump back over same line in opposite direction. Keep a soft bend in knees throughout entire movement. Repeat.

Lateral Hops: Create an imaginary line on the surface you are using. Stand on the side of the imaginary line. While standing straight with slight bend in knees, jump over line in a lateral (side movement), then jump back over same line in opposite direction. Keep a soft bend in knees throughout entire movement. Repeat.

Beginners: Rest at least 1 min, 30 seconds after circuit is complete.

Sets	Performance Time	Repetitions
2-3	20-25 seconds	10-12

Jump rope for 20-30 seconds

Intermediate: Rest 1 minute after entire circuit is complete.

Sets	Performance Time	Repetitions
3-4	25-40 seconds	15-20

Jump rope for 30-45 seconds

Advanced: Rest 30-45 seconds after entire circuit is complete.

Sets	Performance Time	Repetitions
5-6	45 seconds – 1 minute	25-30

Jump rope for 1 minute - 1 minute, 15 seconds

If or when you use cardio machines at the gym, please use the following guidelines to get the most out of your cardio sessions.

CARDIO GUIDELINES

Do not lean on cardio machines: The handles that are provided on each cardio machine are not created for you to lean on. At all times keep body in an upright position with core tight. Leaning on the cardio machine takes away the effectiveness of the exercise by allowing the machines to support your body. Get the most out of every session and don't cheat yourself.

Pay Attention: If you are going to read while doing cardio, make sure your intensity level is sufficient enough to burn calories. Many people read and do not exert enough effort into their cardio. If you want to read, try using the recumbent bike where you can sit and read but still pedal fast.

Get Creative: Using the same cardio machines repeatedly can cause overuse injuries and mental burnout. It is good to mix up your cardio. If you like the bike, why not try adding the elliptical or the stair stepper?

Try Cardio Intervals: Why spend an hour walking slowly on the treadmill when you can spend 30-35 minutes doing intervals and burn more calories? Don't be afraid to try new things - it will shock your body and jump start your metabolism.

GOODBYE LONG

HOURS OF CARDIO!

FIT & FLEXIBLE

We are quickly approaching the lifting chapter and I hope you're anxiously waiting, however before we move to that chapter, I want to talk to you about stretching. Yes, stretching.

One important component to your fitness training program is ensuring you remain flexible in all of your joints. By remaining flexible you lessen your chance of injury and will have a better range of motion to complete your exercises.

Why Stretch?

Some people underestimate the importance and benefits of stretching on a regular basis.

There are numerous benefits to stretching, such as increased range of motion, decreased muscle stiffness and prevention of certain injuries. With so many benefits, stretching should be performed most days of the week following all physical activity. Choosing not to stretch on a regular basis can hinder your range of motion and lead to injuries.

Let's learn the basics of proper stretching.

STRETCHING ESSENTIALS

WHAT IS RANGE OF MOTION (ROM)?

RANGE OF MOTION is the pain free movement around a joint(s). The key word is pain free. As we age, we begin to experience stiffness of our joints and movements become painful as a result of not stretching on a regular basis. Chronic stiffness can lead to limited range of motion, which can lead to improper body mechanics and injuries.

Therefore, in order to avoid these issues, use the following guidelines to stretching and make stretching a regular part of your fitness training program.

STRETCHING GUIDELINES

Never stretch a cold muscle. Imagine placing a rubber band in the freezer for a period of time and then attempting to stretch it. It will not be as pliable cold as it would be at room temperature. Your muscles, ligaments and tendons are similar to a rubber band. The warmer they become, the more pliable they will be. This elasticity will help prevent injuries and increase your range of motion.

Stretch after your workout before complete cool down. Muscles need to have the ability to contract and produce force, therefore stretching too much before your workout could result in less force generated during your lifting. Stretching is used to relax and elongate the muscles, and over stretching prior to resistance training may prevent optimal performance. In order to avoid this, stretch before you reach a cool down state immediately after your training session.

Never bounce. Your body has protective mechanisms which detect the length and force of a stretch. If you stretch your muscles too fast or too far, the body will respond by contracting the muscles. Do not force your body to go beyond its normal range of motion by bouncing or forcing yourself into a stretched position. Forcing your body to go beyond this point can lead to injuries.

Stretch at least three days per week. Regular stretching will provide a greater range of motion to perform Activities of Daily Living (ADLs) such as grocery shopping, gardening and cleaning. Being flexible will, in addition, help you with sports-related performances and lessen chances of injury.

FOLLOW THE F.I.T.T. MODEL FOR STRETCHING

The F.I.T.T. model below teaches you the frequency, intensity, type and time for stretching.

Frequency: At least three days per week, preferably daily and after all physical activity

Intensity: Slow, controlled and not forced. Slowly elongate muscle with low level of force

Type: At least 4-5 stretches per major muscle groups (legs, arms, chest, back)

Time: 15- 30 second holds (static stretching)

The following stretches can be performed after each workout. Remember each stretching guideline and do not force your body beyond its normal range of motion.

UPPER BODY STRETCHES (SHOULDERS, BACK, TRICEPS, CHEST, BICEPS)

TRICEPS STRETCH (STANDING)

Stand in an upright position with a slight bend in knees. Raise your arm over your head and bend your elbow all the way so your hand is behind your neck. Use your opposite arm to stabilize your elbow. Hold for 15-30 seconds. Repeat 3 to 5 times and then perform stretch on the opposite side.

TRICEPS STRETCH (SITTING)

Sit in a chair with body in an upright position, core tight and shoulders back. Raise your arm over your head and bend your elbow all the way so your hand is behind your neck. Use your opposite arm to stabilize your elbow. Hold for 15-30 seconds. Repeat 3 to 5 times and then perform stretch on the opposite side.

SHOULDER ROLLS

Begin sitting or standing with your arms at your sides. Shrug your shoulders up. While your shoulders are in the shrugged position, slowly roll them forward and down. Repeat this movement 5 to 10 times. Then do shoulder shrugs and rolls backward, and repeat this movement 5 to 10 times.

BICEPS STRETCH

Take your arms out to the sides, slightly behind your elbows, with the thumbs up. Rotate your thumbs down and back until they are pointing to the back wall. You will feel a stretch in your biceps. Repeat 3 to 5 times.

REACHING UP AND DOWN

While sitting or standing with your arms at your sides, reach up with one hand toward the ceiling and reach down with the other hand toward the floor. Hold this stretch for 15 to 30 seconds. Repeat 3 to 5 times while alternating arms.

ANTERIOR SHOULDER STRETCH

Stand in a doorway or use a sturdy object (tree, pole) with your right arm out to your side at a 90-degree angle and your elbow flexed to 90 degrees. Place your palm, forearm, and elbow on the door frame (tree/pole). Lean forward through the open door, feeling the stretch in your anterior chest and shoulder. Hold this position for 15 to 30 seconds. Repeat 3 to 5 times and then perform stretch on the opposite side.

UPPER BACK STRETCH

Stand in an upright position, feet together with slight bend in knees. Next, clasps hands in front of body and round back towards floor, pressing arms away from body. You will feel a stretch in the upper part of your back. Keep head in a neutral (head aligned straight) position throughout movement. Hold position. Repeat 3 to 5 times.

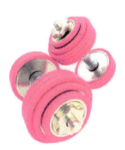

FIT JEWEL

Choosing not to stretch on a regular basis can hinder your range of motion and lead to injuries.

LOWER BODY STRETCHES (GLUTES, HAMSTRINGS AND CALVES)

GLUTEAL (BUTTOCKS) STRETCH

Sit in a chair or lie on your back. Flex (bend) one knee toward your chest and place your hands around the front of your knee, pulling the knee up towards the shoulder of the same side and you will feel the stretch in your gluteal (buttocks) area. Hold position for 15 to 30 seconds. Repeat 3 to 5 times and then perform stretch on the opposite side.

HIP FLEXOR (HIPS) STRETCH

Stand with your hands grasping a chair or sturdy object (tree). With your left foot supporting your body weight and right leg extended back, push your pelvis forward with your torso in the upright position, you will feel the stretch in the front of your hip. Hold this position for 15 to 30 seconds. Repeat 3 to 5 times and then perform stretch on the opposite side.

HAMSTRING STRETCH (STANDING)

While standing, place one foot forward on a bench or step with knee slightly bent. While supporting most of your weight on the other foot, lean forward at the waist with arms reaching toward your toes, you will feel the stretch in the back of your thigh (hamstrings). Hold this position for 15 to 30 seconds. Repeat 3 to 5 times and then perform stretch on the opposite side.

HAMSTRING STRETCH (LYING DOWN)

Lie on your back, place one leg in the air, while opposite leg rests on the floor. With slight bend in knee, position hands underneath your knee and gently move knee towards chest, you will feel the stretch in your hamstring. Hold this position for 15 to 30 seconds. Repeat 3 to 5 times and then perform stretch on the opposite side.

QUADRICEPS (FRONT PART OF LEG) STRETCH

Standing with your right hand grasping a chair for stability, hold your left ankle behind you with your left hand, pulling it upward and backward and feeling the stretch in the front of your thigh. Hold this position for 15 to 30 seconds. Repeat 3 to 5 times and then perform stretch on the opposite side.

CALF STRETCH (BENT KNEE)

Standing with your arms stretched in front of you and hands on a wall, support your weight on the right foot with the right knee slightly bent while placing your left foot behind you with the heel on the ground and the knee slightly bent. Lean forward, you will feel the stretch in your calf. Hold for 15 to 30 seconds. Repeat 3 to 5 times. Perform this stretch on the opposite side.

CALF STRETCH (STRAIGHT KNEE)

Standing with your arms stretched in front of you and hands on a wall, support your weight on your right foot with knee slightly bent while placing your left foot behind you with the heel on the ground and the knee straight. Lean forward, you will feel the stretch in your calf. Hold for 15 to 30 seconds. Repeat 3 to 5 times. Perform this stretch on the opposite side.

Put It All Together

Before moving on to the amazing exercises in the next chapter, take a moment and familiarize yourself with how to set up your weight lifting program. Consider this a roadmap from start to finish!

Step 1). Determine Your Days: Determine which days of the week you are going to devote to your workouts (ex. Monday, Wednesday, and Friday). On the days that you perform your resistance training perform at least 30 minutes of cardio or more time your current fitness condition allows you.

If or when you only have an hour to workout, split your time doing 30 minutes of resistance training and 30 minutes of cardiovascular exercise including a general warm-up. If you only have 30 minutes for cardiovascular activities, I recommend doing intervals which consists of doing a high level burst of activity, followed by rest for a short period of time before going back to the high level activity (Ex. Sprint for 1 minute, recover by walking for 30 seconds).

Step 2). Determine Which Body Part(s): Once you have determined which days of the week you're going to train, you will then determine which muscle(S) group (s) you're going to train. If you're a beginner it is recommended that you perform a total body routine which allows you to perform at least 2 exercises for each major muscle group. Performing a total body routine, places less stress on any particular muscle group which will assist you in possible injuries and early burnout.

Intermediate and advanced individuals may exercise one or two muscle groups at a time, 3-4 days per week allowing at least 48 hours of rest between each muscle group for recovery.

Step 3). Have Your Plan Ready: Prior to arriving to the gym, know which muscle groups you're going to train and what exercises you're going to perform to train them. Once you have completed your general warm-up go straight to performing your resistance training exercises. Stay focused and move from one exercise to another in a circuit fashion if your current fitness level allows you to accomplish this. Don't rest any longer than 60-90 seconds after one set of exercises or no longer than 90 seconds after a complete circuit.

Step 4). Warm-Up Properly: Prior to each workout session perform a warm-up for at least 5-10 minutes of light to moderately light physical activity. This could mean walking on the treadmill or cycling on the bike. The warm-up is essential in increasing your core temperature and prepares your body for your workout. NEVER skip a warm-up; doing so can increase your risk of injury which can lead to chronic issues if left untreated.

Step 5). Cardio Time: Once you have completed your resistance training routine, go straight to your cardiovascular activity. By this time your core temperature has been raised your body is ready to perform your cardio.

Step 6). Stretch Please: Once you have completed your cardio, stretch each large muscle group in what is known as a static hold stretch for 15-30 seconds. At all times only stretch as far as your body naturally will allow you to. Do not bounce while you're stretching and do not stretch cold muscles! Perform at least 1-2 stretches per muscle group most if not all days of the week.

WORKOUT NUTRITION GUIDELINES:

- **PRE- WORKOUT:** Solid Foods: For optimal performance ensure you are eating at least 2 hours prior to your training session. Therefore prior to your workout session consume a good source of protein and complex carbohydrate such a peanut butter and jelly sandwich with a glass of Almond Milk. Carbohydrates are your bodies' main fuel source and when consumed with a healthy source of protein, can sustain your energy levels throughout your workouts. (Ex. A peanut butter and banana sandwich, protein drink and 1 piece of fruit). If you don't want a solid try a liquid and consume at least 1 hour prior to workout. This can consist of a protein drink with frozen fruit.

- **MID-WORKOUT:** If you're training at a high intensity beyond 1 hour it may be essential to replenish your glycogen (sugar) stores with an intra-workout drink such Gatorade or PowerAde. Drink only when needed due to the amount of sugar found in these drinks.

- **POST WORKOUT:** Within 30 minutes from the completion of your workout, consume a healthy source of protein and carbohydrates.

HYDRATION:

DRINK WATER BEFORE, during and after each workout. Water assists your body in temperature regulation during and after workouts. Don't forget to stay hydrated, dehydration can affect performance and cause cramps.

TECHNIQUE GUIDELINES:

- At all times maintain proper form and never jeopardize form in order to make increases in the amount of weight you desire to lift. The key to progress is to perform EACH movement with proper form with an amount of weight that is appropriate to your current fitness level.

- Allow at least 24-48 hours between each training session of each muscle group in order to avoid overtraining and to recover properly. You may experience soreness which may peak 48-72 hours after your training session. This is referred to as Delayed Onset Muscle Soreness or DOMS. This is a natural effect of exercise however, listen to your bodies signals. If you remain sore for longer than 72 hours you may need to drop your amount of weight, sets and repetitions and rest for longer periods of time after your workouts.

It's Lifting Time!

I f you're a beginner to exercise, it is essential to slowly incorporate weight training into your fitness training program. Therefore it is recommended to do three days of weight training per week on non-consecutive days (Monday, Wednesday, and Friday). Doing more than three days per week at the beginning of your fitness training program may result in mental burnout and injuries.

It is also recommended to incorporate cardiovascular exercise on the same day as your resistance training. On the days in which you choose to perform both resistance training and cardiovascular activities, perform your resistance training exercises first followed by your cardiovascular activities. Later in this chapter you will find a step-by-step guide teaching you how to flow throughout your entire workout from start to finish.

Intermediate and advanced level individuals, you can incorporate resistance training five days per week for your fitness training program. At this stage, you have the strength to perform more volume. In addition to your resistance training, perform cardiovascular activities five days a week, allowing at least 48 hours of rest in between each muscle group. The body's muscle fibers are broken down when you resistance train, therefore, rest time is essential in assisting your body in recovery and repair.

Before you begin the following exercises to sculpt your curves, identify your current fitness training level. Identifying your current fitness training level will assist you in choosing the proper amount of sets, repetitions and rest time for each exercise.

IDENTIFY YOUR FITNESS TRAINING LEVEL

IDENTIFY WHETHER OR not you're beginner, intermediate or advanced level. Based on your training level, determine how many sets and repetitions you will perform for each exercise.

Beginner: No previous experience with resistance training or recreational activities.

Intermediate: Train at least 3 days per week, including cardiovascular activities.

Advanced: An athlete or you have more than a year experience with resistance training. Train at least 4-5 days per week.

SETS AND REPETITIONS

BELOW YOU FIND the amount of sets and repetitions that you will perform based on your current fitness level.

Beginner: Perform: 2 sets per exercise for 10-12 repetitions using light weight (5-8 lbs.). Perform modified version (MV) for each exercise that isn't within your current fitness level.

Intermediate: Perform: 3 sets per exercise for 12-15 repetitions each using moderate weight (10-15 lbs.).

Advanced: Perform 3-5 sets per exercise for 6-8 repetitions for strength and 12-15 repetitions for tone. Use moderate to heavier weight (15 lbs. or more).

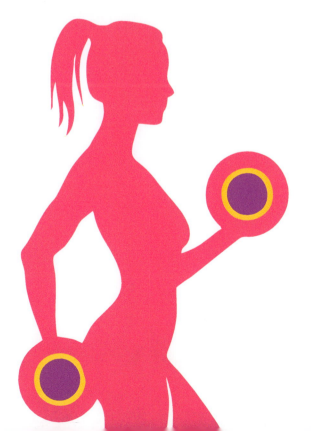

Upper Body Exercises

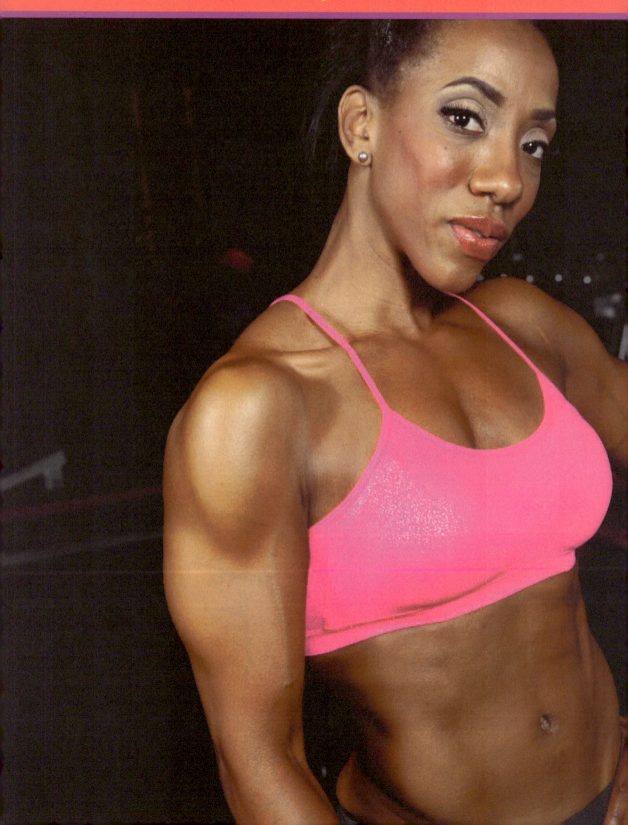

TIGHTEN, FIRM AND TONE

A STRONG AND toned upper body not only looks great for the warmer months when sleeveless shirts and swimsuits are worn, but toned arms are also great for assisting you in activities of daily living such as picking up your children, carrying groceries and being able lift and carry your laundry. Research has shown that after the age of 30 women begin to lose muscle tissue by 3 to 5 percent per decade. A loss of muscle tissue can lead to diminished mobility and strength in the aging process, therefore it is essential to incorporate resistance training into your normal fitness regimen on a regular basis.

The following exercises in this chapter will help you sculpt and tone your upper body without adding a bulky appearance. Discover your skill level and perform the exercises prescribed to you. If you are a beginner, listen to your body and only perform the amount of sets and repetitions that feel appropriate for you. Intermediate and advanced levels - don't be afraid to safely push your body by adding extra resistance and increasing your repetitions.

HELLO SEXY ARMS AND HELLO SUMMERTIME!

CHEST EXERCISES

Movement Tip: To avoid injury, keep core contracted throughout entire movement. Doing so will keep body aligned and lessen the chance of injury to your back.

BEGINNER LEVEL

Exercise	Sets	Repetitions
One-Arm Med Ball Pushups *Modified Version	2-3	4-6
Single-Legged Chest Press	2-3	8-10 each arm
Physio-ball Chest Press	2-3	10-12 each arm
Resistance Band Flyes	2-3	10-12

INTERMEDIATE LEVEL

Exercise	Sets	Repetitions
One-Arm Med Ball Pushups	3-4	15-20
Single-Legged Chest Press	3-4	15-20 each arm
Physio-ball Chest Press	3-4	15-20 each arm
Physio-ball Pushups	3-4	10-15
Resistance Band Flyes	3-4	12-15

ADVANCED LEVEL

Exercise	Sets	Repetitions
One-Arm Med Ball Pushups	4-5	15
Single-Legged Chest Press	4-5	15
Physio-ball Chest Press	4-5	15 each arm
One-Arm Med Ball Pushups	4-5	15
Resistance Band Flyes	4-5	15-20

ONE-ARM MED BALL PUSHUPS

Targeted Muscles: chest, triceps

Set Up: Kneel on the ground with hands positioned shoulder width apart, one hand resting on med ball with other hand placed on ground. From kneeling position, extend arms and legs.

Action: In a slow and controlled manner, bend your elbows and lower your body until arms form a 90-degree angle. Hold for a count and then extend your arms and push body back to starting position. Complete set and then switch arms.

Movement Tip: To avoid back injury, keep core tight and body in straight position. Do not drop hips.

*Modified Version: Perform exercise on your knees.

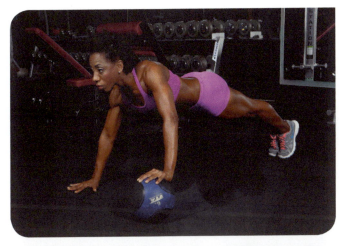

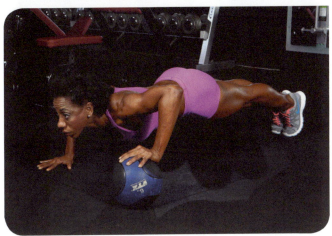

PHYSIO-BALL PUSHUPS

Targeted Muscles: chest, triceps

Set Up: Place stability ball in front of body. Slowly roll your body onto the ball until your shins rest on ball. Your arms are positioned shoulder width apart with lower body and core tight. Keep slight bend in elbows.

Action: In a slow and controlled manner, bend elbows and slowly lower body until your arms form a 90- degree angle. Hold for a count and then extend arms to return body to starting position. Repeat movement until set is complete.

Movement Tip: To avoid injury, keep core tight throughout entire movement.

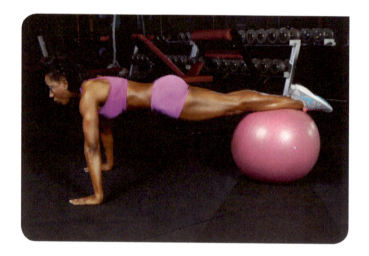

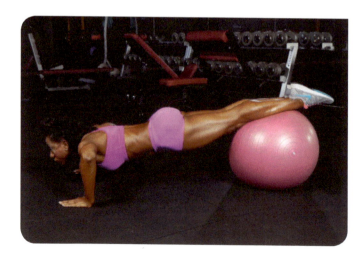

SINGLE-LEGGED CHEST PRESS

Targeted Muscles: glutes, hamstrings, chest, triceps

Set Up: Lay on back with both feet on ground, knees bent with arms bent holding dumbbells at chest level.

Action: In an upward movement, slowly bridge up on one leg, with opposite leg elevated off ground. Once lower body is off ground, press dumbbell upward until arms are fully extended. Hold for a count and then bring body back to starting position. Complete set and then switch to opposite arm and leg.

*Modified Version: Keep both feet on ground. Maintain body in bridged position.

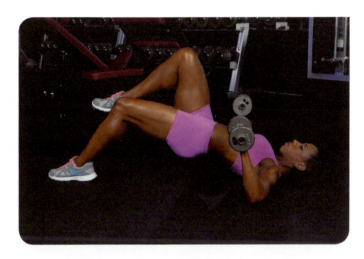

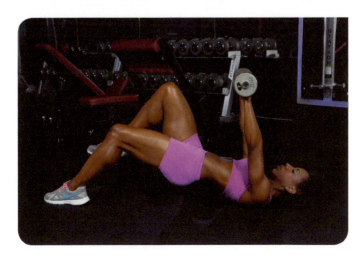

PHYSIO-BALL CHEST PRESS

Targeted Muscles: chest, triceps

Set Up: Position body on a stability ball with a pair of dumbbells in both hands with feet positioned apart. In a slow and controlled manner, slowly walk your feet away from the ball until your upper back rests on stability ball. Elbows are bent with dumbbells facing inward with hips parallel to floor and feet positioned slightly apart.

Action: In a slow and controlled manner, slowly lower weight to sides of upper chest until slight stretch is felt in chest or shoulder. Hold for a count and then slowly extend arms to starting position without locking elbows. Keep core engaged and hips elevated in order to maintain form throughout entire movement.

Movement Tip: Keep hips and core contracted.

*Modified Version: Drop hips to mid-level. Keep core contracted at all times.

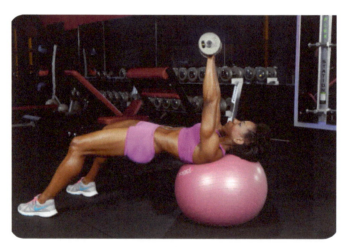

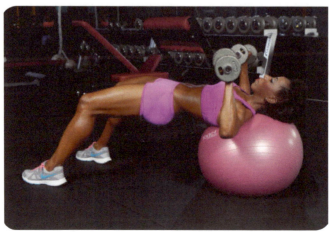

CHEST PRESS WITH BRIDGE

Targeted Muscles: glutes, hamstring and chest

Set Up: Lay on your back with knees bent, feet flat on floor, elbows bent while holding medicine ball at chest level.

Action: In a slow and controlled manner, lift body off mat by squeezing glutes and hamstrings in an upward movement (bridge), while keeping ball near chest. Once hips are off ground, extend arms and press ball towards ceiling. When balls returns, catch ball with slight bend in elbows. Bring lower body down from bridge movement and repeat entire movement.

Movement Tip: Find a focal point on the ceiling when tossing the ball. This will allow to you to remain consistent with pressing the ball upward and catching it in the same spot.

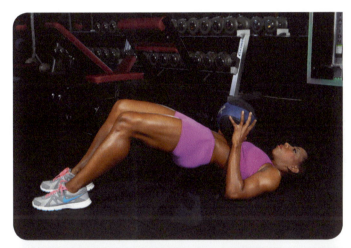

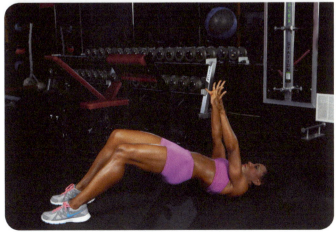

AROUND THE WORLD

Targeted Muscles: chest, triceps

Set Up: Begin in pushup position with hands shoulder width apart, body in a straight line, core and lower body tight.

Action: In a slow and controlled manner, slowly bend your elbows and lower body until you reach a 90-degree angle. Hold for a count and then extend your arms and return to starting position. While in starting pushup position, lift right arm and rotate arm across body and hold for a count. Bring arm down. Perform another pushup and then repeat lift with opposite arm.

***Modified Version:** Perform exercise on knees.

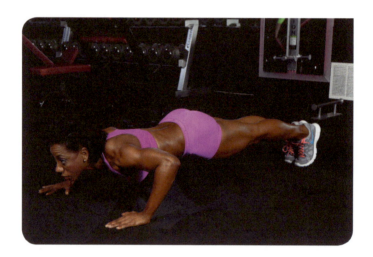

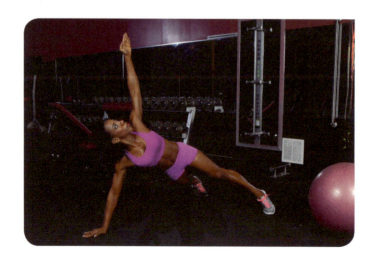

RESISTANCE BANDS FLYES

Targeted Muscles: chest, triceps

Set Up: While in a standing position, with chest up shoulder blades back and slight bend in knees, grab resistant band and place behind the back of your shoulders. Once band is placed behind shoulders place a bend in elbows with arms extended out to the side of your body.

Action: With a slight bend in elbows, squeeze chest muscles together and bring arms together with palms facing one another. Hold for account and bring arms back to starting position. Repeat until set is complete.

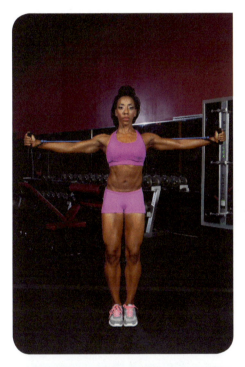 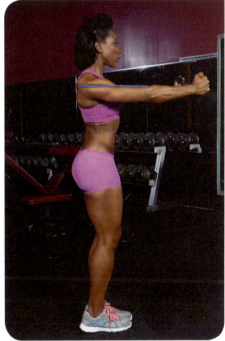

FIT JEWEL

Using resistance training bands is a non-expensive and fun way to get fit at the gym, at home or while you travel. If you travel often, packing a resistance training band in your suitcase will allow you to stay fit on the go. You can get fit and creative with resistance training bands!

BACK EXERCISES

Movement Tip: Keep core contracted while performing each exercise. This will keep body aligned and lessen the chance of injury to your back.

BEGINNER LEVEL

Exercise	Sets	Repetitions
Seated Resistance Band Rows	2-3	10-12
One-Arm Row	2-3	10-12
Two-Arm Row *Modified Version	2-3	10-12

INTERMEDIATE LEVEL

Exercise	Sets	Repetitions
Seated Resistance Band Rows	3-4	15-20
One-Arm Row	3-4	15-20
Two-Arm Row	3-4	15-20

ADVANCED LEVEL

Exercise	Sets	Repetitions
Seated Resistance Band Rows	4-5	8-15
One-Arm Row	4-5	8-15
Two-Arm Row	4-5	8-15

SEATED RESISTANCE BAND ROWS

Targeted Muscles: back, chest

Set Up: While in a seated position, shoulder back, core engaged and chest up, with knees bent and heels on the ground, place resistance band under the base of your shoe, grasping both handles with arms fully extended.

Action: In a slow and controlled manner, bring elbows back by squeezing shoulder blades together. Hold for a count and repeat entire movement until set is complete.

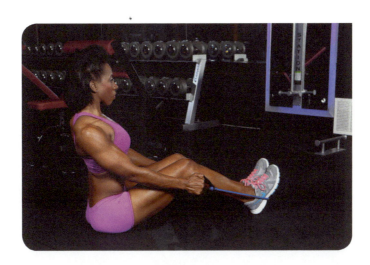

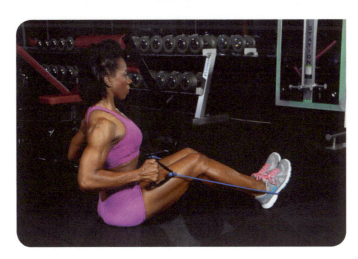

ONE-ARM ROW

Targeted Muscles: back, core

Set Up: Begin by standing in a split stance, with one foot staggered in front of the other. Place a slight bend in knees, arm holding dumbbells in front of body with slight lean in torso.

Action: In a slow and controlled manner with core engaged, bring elbow back by squeezing your shoulder blade. Hold for a count and then extend arm back to starting position. Complete movements until set is complete and then switch arms.

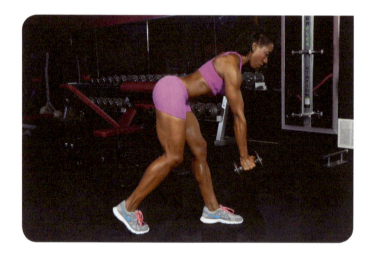

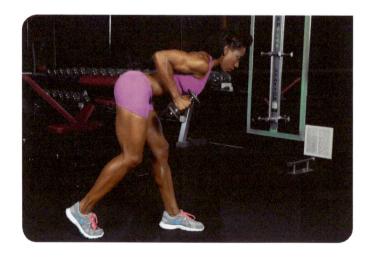

TWO-ARM ROW

Targeted Muscles: back, core

Set Up: Begin by standing in a split stance, with one foot staggered in front of the other. Place a slight bend in knees, lean in torso, with arms extended in front of body holding dumbbells.

Action: In a slow and controlled manner with core engaged, bring elbows back by squeezing your shoulder blades together. Hold for a count and then extend arms back to starting position. Complete movement until set is complete.

*Modified Version: Keep torso forward, but keep back leg on the ground.

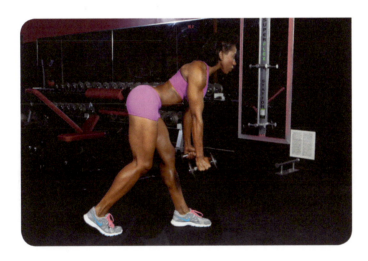

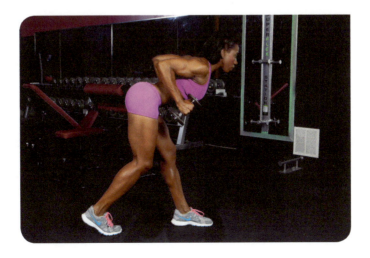

SHOULDER EXERCISES

Movement Tip: Keep core contracted while performing each exercise. This will keep body aligned and lessen the chance of injury to your back.

BEGINNER LEVEL

Exercise	Sets	Repetitions
Core Shoulder Lifts *Modified Version	2-3	8-10
Front Shoulder Raises	2-3	10-12
Lateral Shoulder Raises	2-3	10-12
Rear Shoulder Raises	2-3	10-12

INTERMEDIATE LEVEL

Exercise	Sets	Repetitions
Core Shoulder Lifts	3-4	15-20
Front Shoulder Raises	3-4	15-20
Lateral Shoulder Raises	3-4	15-20
Rear Shoulder Raises	3-4	15-20

ADVANCED LEVEL

Exercise	Sets	Repetitions
Core Shoulder Lifts*	4	12-15
Front Shoulder Raises	4-5	8-15
Lateral Shoulder Raises	4-5	8-15
Rear Shoulder Raises	4-5	8-15

*Use a heavier medicine ball around 8-10 lbs. for added resistance

CORE SHOULDER LIFTS

Targeted Muscles: anterior deltoids (front shoulder), core

Set Up: Position body on a mat with feet flat on floor, knees bent, chest up and arms extended in front of body while holding medicine ball.

Action: With core tight, in a slow and controlled manner, slightly lean back and raise feet about 2 inches off ground (Advanced level can raise feet higher). Once stabilized in position, lift arms in an upward position. Hold for a count, and then bring arms down. Repeat movement.

Movement Tip: Keep core tight and chest up to avoid rounding back while performing movement.

*Modified Version: Keep both feet on ground.

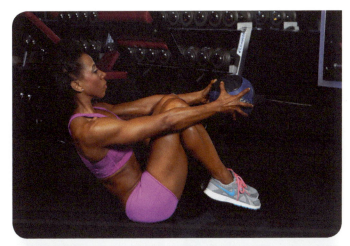

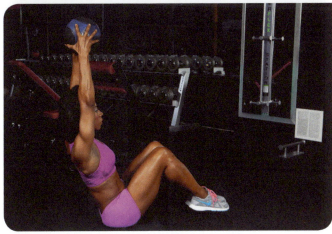

KEEP YOUR CORE TIGHT!

FRONT SHOULDER RAISES

Targeted Muscles: anterior deltoids (front shoulder)

Set up: Stand in an upright position, feet positioned together or apart, core engaged with slight bend in knees. Dumbbells held in a neutral (palms facing inward towards your body) position in your hands.

Action: In a slow and controlled manner lift dumbbells in an upward movement raising arms until they reach eye level with palms facing each other. Hold for a count and then return hands back to starting position.

Movement tip: Keep slight bend in knees throughout the entire movement and don't allow body to swing as you move the dumbbells away from your body. Keep core engaged and feet anchored to ground in order to avoid swinging movement.

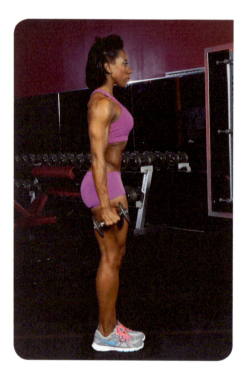 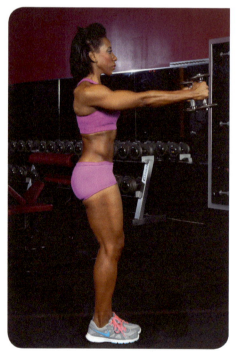

FIT JEWEL

Hello summer and short sleeve shirts!

LATERAL SHOULDER RAISES

Targeted Muscles: lateral deltoids (middle of shoulder)

Set Up: Stand with your feet together, knees slightly bent, while holding dumbbells facing inward towards your hips.

Action: With a slight bend in elbows, in a slow and controlled manner, lift arms in a lateral position (lateral means away from the mid-line of your body) until arms are parallel to the floor. Hold for a count and then lower arms back to starting position. Repeat movement until set is complete.

Movement Tip: Do not bring arms too high. As a reference point, you should be able to see the back of your hands in your peripheral view. If you can't see your hands, you're lifting too high. Raising arms to high releases tension off shoulder and places stress on other muscles. Do not arch back throughout movement.

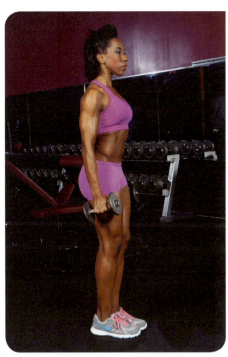 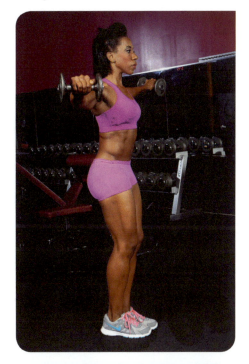

FIT JEWEL
Toned shoulders look great regardless of what you wear, therefore don't forget to incorporate shoulder exercises into your fitness training program.

REAR SHOULDER RAISES

Targeted Muscles: rear deltoids, core

Set Up: Begin with feet together, knees bent, torso forward with arms extended in front of body holding dumbbells facing inward towards body.

Action: With a slight bend in elbows, in a slow and controlled manner, lift arms away from body in an arching movement by squeezing shoulder blades together. Hold for a count and then lower arms back to starting position. Repeat movement until set is complete.

Movement Tip: Keep knees bent and core tight.

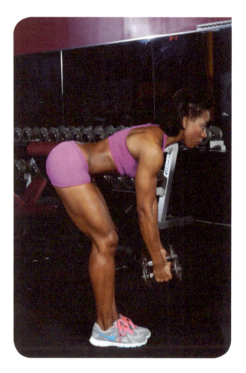 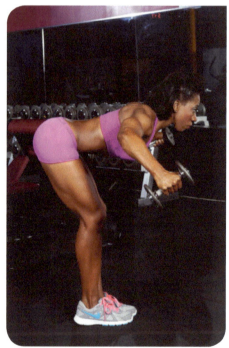

FIT JEWEL

Nice toned shoulders are great for the winter, summer or anytime of the year!

BICEP EXERCISES

Movement Tip: Keep core contracted while performing each exercise. This will keep body aligned and lessen the chance of injury to your back.

BEGINNER LEVEL

Exercise	Sets	Repetitions
Kneeling Physio-ball Curls	2-3	8-10
Single-Legged Bicep Curls *Modified Version	2-3	8-10
Split Stance Hammer Curls	2-3	8-10
Resistance Bands Curls	2-3	8-10

INTERMEDIATE LEVEL

Exercise	Sets	Repetitions
Kneeling Physio-ball Curls	3-4	10-12
Single-Legged Bicep Curls	3-4	10-12
Split Stance Bicep Curls	3-4	10-12
Resistance Bands Curls	3-4	10-12

ADVANCED LEVEL

Exercise	Sets	Repetitions
Kneeling Physio-ball Curls	4-5	12-15
Single-Legged Bicep Curls	4-5	12-15
Split Stance Bicep Curls	4-5	12-15
Resistance Bands Curls	4-5	12-15

KNEELING PHYSIO-BALL CURLS

Targeted Muscles: biceps

Set Up: Kneel down in front of physio-ball with elbows positioned on ball, with palms facing upward while holding dumbbells along with core engaged.

Action: In a slow and controlled manner, squeeze biceps and bring down dumbbells towards your shoulders, keeping elbows close to body. Hold for a count and then extend arms without full extension of elbow back to starting position. Repeat movement until set is complete.

Movement Tip: Keep core tight to avoid hurting your lower back and if you experience knee problems, place a mat or towel under knees.

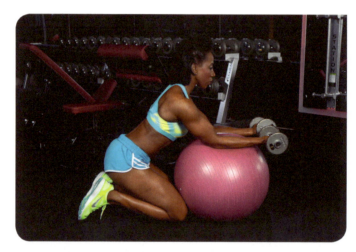

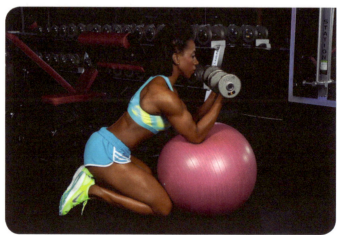

BE AWARE OF YOUR POSTURE AT ALL TIMES!

SINGLE-LEGGED BICEP CURLS

Targeted Muscles: biceps, core

Set Up: Stand with both feet together, slight bend in knees. Arms positioned by side, with palms facing away from your body while holding dumbbells.

Action: In a slow and controlled manner, slowly lift one leg off ground. Once stabilized, with elbow locked near side, curl dumbbell upward by squeezing biceps. Hold for a count and then lower arms back to starting position without locking out elbows. Repeat movement until set is complete and then switch leg.

Movement Tip: Slowly bring arms down without fully extending them.

*Modified Version: Keep both feet on ground or bring foot slightly off the ground.

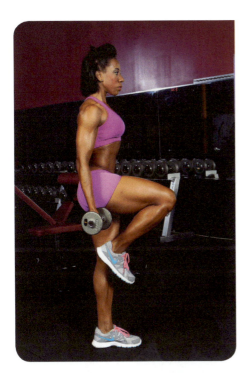 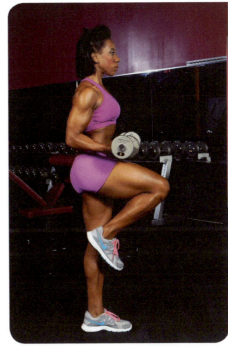

FIT JEWEL

While standing on one leg, keep core engaged this will help you keep your balance.

SPLIT STANCE HAMMER CURLS

Targeted Muscles: biceps

Set Up: In an upright position stagger feet evenly positioning body weight on front and back legs, with shoulders back, core engaged while holding dumbbells in a neutral position (palms facing towards your body), with slight bend in elbows.

Action: In a slow and controlled manner, slowly squeeze biceps and bring dumbbells towards your shoulder while keeping elbows positioned close to your body. Hold for a count and then return hands to starting position without fully extending arms. Repeat movement until set is complete.

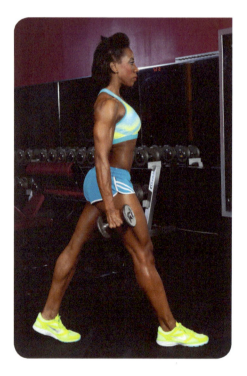 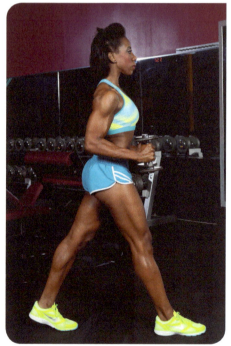

FIT JEWEL

Never jeopardize form for weight. If you can't properly lift the weight you're using, decrease the amount of weight.

RESISTANCE BANDS CURLS

Targeted Muscles: biceps

Set Up: Place resistance band underneath both feet creating enough space to create equal resistance on handles. Once band is placed under feet, stand in an upright position with shoulders back, core engaged, slight bend in knees and palms facing upward with resistance band in both hands.

Action: In a slow and controlled manner with elbows close to body, squeeze biceps and bring hands towards shoulders, hold for a count and then return hands to starting position without fully extending arms.

Movement Tip: Keep a slight bend in knees at all times in order to avoid placing stress on your lower back. When performing movement, do not allow elbows to move away from the body, doing so will place less stress on biceps.

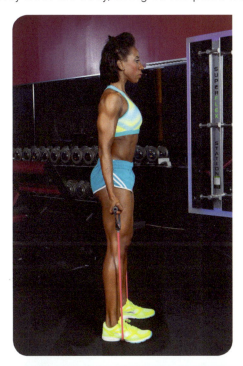 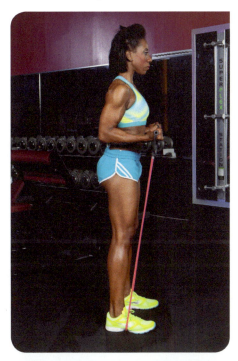

FIT JEWEL

Keep elbows locked into your side in order to fully make the biceps work.

TRICEPS EXERCISES

Movement Tip: Keep core contracted while performing each exercise. This will keep body aligned and lessen the chance of injury to your back.

BEGINNER LEVEL

Exercise	Sets	Repetitions
Resistance Band Extensions	1-2	8-10
Standing Triceps Kickbacks	1-2	8-10
Seated Overhead Triceps Extensions *Modified Version	1-2	8-10

INTERMEDIATE LEVEL

Exercise	Sets	Repetitions
Resistance Band Extensions	2-3	10-12
Standing Triceps Kickbacks	2-3	10-12
Seated Overhead Triceps Extensions	2-3	10-12
Pyramid Pushups	2-3	10-12

ADVANCED LEVEL

Exercise	Sets	Repetitions
Resistance Band Extensions	3-4	12-15
Standing Triceps Kickbacks	3-4	12-15
Seated Overhead Triceps Extensions	3-4	12-15
Physio-ball Triceps Pushups	3-4	12-15

RESISTANCE BAND EXTENSIONS

Targeted Muscles: Triceps

Set Up: Place resistance band underneath the back of your foot and then stand in an upright position staggering feet evenly in order to position body weight on front and back legs. Shoulders back, core engaged while holding resistance band in hand with elbow bent.

Action: In a slow and controlled manner, contract core and fully extend arm by squeezing triceps without locking out your elbow. Hold for a count and then return arm back to starting position. Repeat movement until set is complete and then switch your arm and foot.

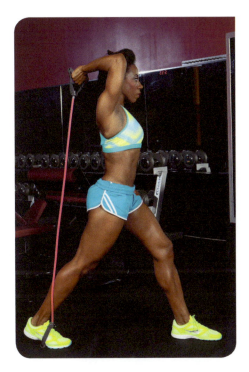
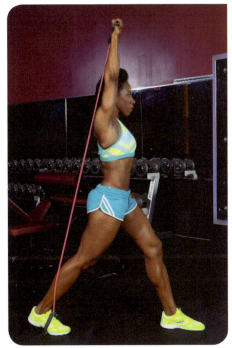

FIT JEWEL

Performing these exercises will give you the confidence to wave goodbye!

ONE-ARM TRICEPS EXTENSIONS

Targeted Muscles: triceps, core

Set Up: Place body in push up position, with hands positioned shoulder width apart. Legs spread apart to form a V with dumbbells in front of body.

Action: While contracting core, slowly grab dumbbell off floor and lift right arm off ground, tucking right elbow at side. Once elbow is tucked into side, in a slow and controlled manner, extend arm without locking out. Repeat movement until set is complete and then switch arms. Complete set with opposite arm.

Movement Tip: To avoid back injuries, keep core contracted throughout entire movement.

*Modified version: Perform on knees.

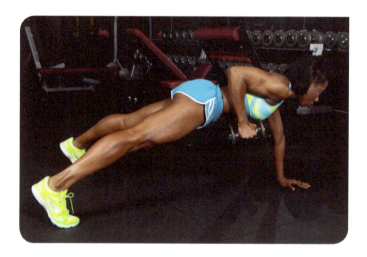

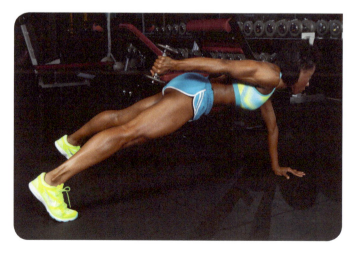

PHYSIO-BALL TRICEPS PUSHUPS

Targeted Muscles: triceps, core

Set Up: In a slow and controlled manner, roll body forward onto stability ball until shins are resting on ball. Hands are positioned closer than shoulder width, with slight bend in elbows.

Action: In a slow and controlled manner, bend elbows in a hinge movement and lower body about 2-4 inches from the ground. Hold for a count and then extend arms to return body to starting position. Repeat movement until set is complete.

Movement Tip: To help balance on ball, keep core contracted and lower body aligned.

*Modified Version: Do not use ball, instead use mat and perform exercise on knees. Keep core tight throughout entire movement.

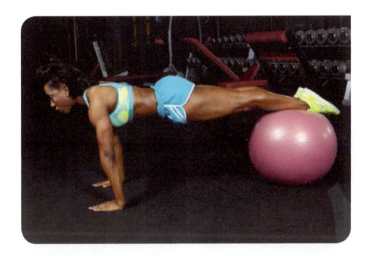

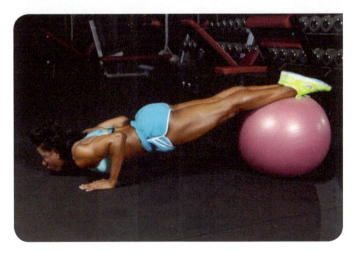

STANDING TRICEPS KICKBACKS

Targeted Muscles: triceps, core

Set Up: Stand with feet together, slight bend in knees. Torso forward and elbows tucked into side of body while holding dumbbells in a supinated position (hands facing upwards towards your body).

Action: In a slow and controlled manner, extend your arms by squeezing your triceps. Hold for a count and then bring arms back to starting position. Repeat movement until set is complete.

Movement Tip: Fully extend arms without locking elbows.

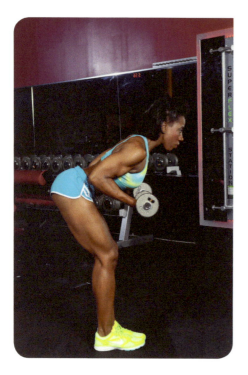 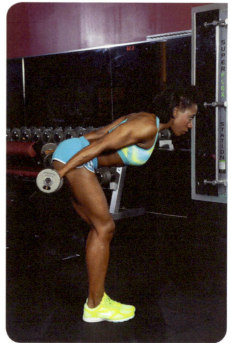

FIT JEWEL

To avoid overuse injuries at the elbow joint, don't lock out elbows on triceps exercises.

PYRAMID PUSHUPS

Targeted Muscles: triceps, core and chest

Set Up: Start with body in a pushup position, hands are positioned close together with index fingers and thumbs touching to form a diamond. Lower body and core remain aligned and contracted.

Action: In a slow and controlled manner, bend elbows and lower body parallel to floor. Once arms are positioned at 90-degrees, stop movement. Hold for a count and then extend arms to return to starting position. Repeat movement until set is complete. Do not lockout elbows when returning to starting position.

Movement Tip: To avoid back injuries, keep core tight throughout entire movement.

*Modified Version: Perform exercise on knees.

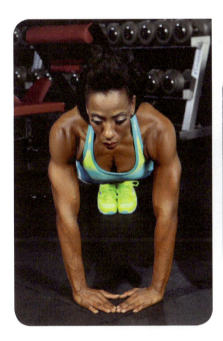 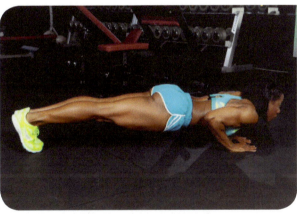

FIT JEWEL

Many women have weaker upper bodies, but performing this exercise will help improve your upper body strength and tone your arms.

SEATED OVERHEAD TRICEPS EXTENSIONS

Targeted Muscles: triceps, core

Set Up: Place body on a stability ball while holding dumbbells. In a slow and controlled manner, walk your feet away from ball until your upper back rests on stability ball. Hips parallel to the floor with arms extended holding dumbbells.

Action: While maintaining balance on stability ball, in a slow and controlled manner, bend elbows and lower weight until your elbows are fully bent. Hold for a count and then extend arms back to starting position. Repeat movement until set is complete.

*Movement Tip: Extend arms without locking elbows.

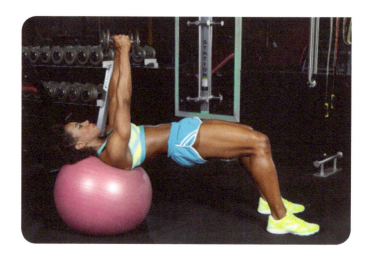

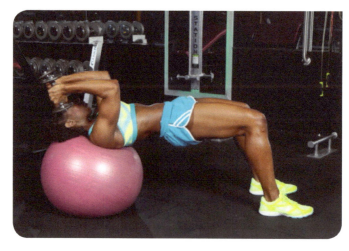

STRAIGHT ARM EXTENSIONS

Targeted Muscles: triceps, core

Set up: Stand in an upright position with body facing towards triceps extension attachment either on a Smith Machine or Universal Cable System. Shoulder blades back, slight bend in knees, core engaged and hand positioned in supinated position (palms facing upward).

Action: In a slow and controlled manner fully extend arm by squeezing triceps. Extend arm without locking elbow. Hold for a count and then return arm back to starting position. Repeat movement until set is complete and then switch arms.

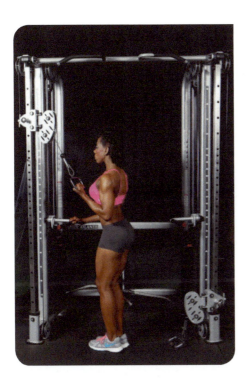 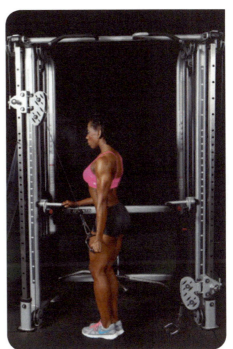

FIT JEWEL

Using the cable machine is a great way to add variety into your resistance training program.

PHYSIO-BALL OVERHEAD TRICEPS EXTENSIONS

Targeted Muscles: triceps, core

Set Up: Sit on physio-ball with slight bend in knees, feet flat on ground, core engaged, shoulders back and arms extended holding dumbbells.

Action: While maintaining stability on ball, in a slow and controlled manner, bend elbows and lower weight until your hands are behind your head. Hold for a count and then extend arms back to starting position. Repeat movement until set is complete.

Movement Tip: Extend arms without locking elbows out.

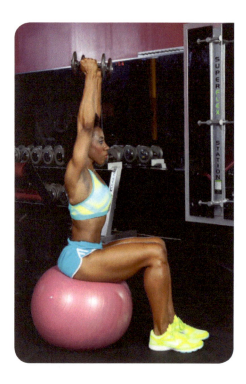 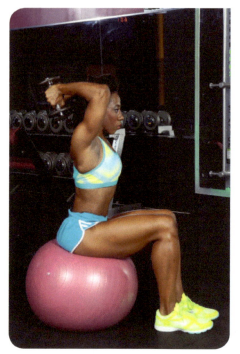

FIT JEWEL

Performing exercises on an unstable object such as the physio-ball is a great way to build core strength and balance.

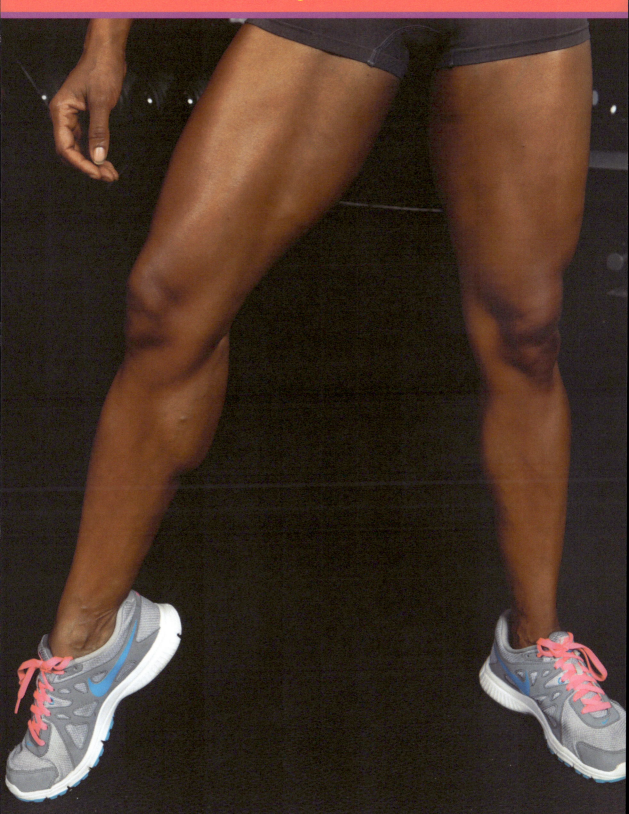

HIPS, GLUTES AND THIGHS, OH MY!

Have you ever turned around and looked at your backside and thought, "I wish my backside was firmer?" Whether you are 26 or 46, at some point in time most women have made this statement to themselves. The backside, or the glutes and the thighs, for many women are the hardest and most challenging area to firm, tighten and tone. Women naturally carry more body fat in these areas, and as a result find it harder to see the tone they desire. Do you find it hard to tone these areas of your body?

If this is you, the exercises on the following pages are designed not only to help you look great in your favorite jeans, but the following exercises are also designed to help you keep your legs strong enough to run, bike, dance and perform all other activities of living. A firmer backside and toned legs are only a few squats away, what are you waiting for?

TONED LEGS NOT ONLY LOOK GREAT IN A PAIR OF JEANS OR SHORTS, THEY ARE ALSO GREAT FOR JUMPING AND OTHER SPORTING ACTIVITIES

LOWER BODY EXERCISES

Movement Tip: Keep core contracted while performing each exercise. This will keep body aligned and lessen the chance of injury to your back.

Exercise Tip: In order to make lunges and squats more difficult, add dumbbells.

BEGINNER LEVEL

Exercise	Sets	Repetitions
Reverse Lunges	1-2	10-12
Hamstring Blast	1-2	10-12
Hamstring Reach	1-2	10-12
Frog Lifts	1-2	10-12

INTERMEDIATE LEVEL

Exercise	Sets	Repetitions
Squat Kicks	2-3	12-15
Lunge Ups	2-3	12-15
Single Legged Bridges	2-3	12-15
Frog Lifts	2-3	12-15

ADVANCED LEVEL

Exercise	Sets	Repetitions
Squat Kicks	3-4	15-20
Frog Lifts	3-4	15-20
Single Legged Bridges	3-4	15-20
Hamstring Reaches	3-4	15-20
Lateral Lunges	3-4	15-20

REVERSE LUNGES

Targeted Muscles: quadriceps, glutes and hamstrings

Set Up: Stand with feet together, slight bend in knees with hands resting on hips or placed in front of body.

Action: With chest up and core tight, in a slow and controlled manner, step back with one leg, creating a wide stance between your front and back leg. Keep a slight bend in both knees without knees going over toes. Your back knee approaches the ground but never touches the ground. Hold for a count and push off back leg, bring back leg forward to starting position. Repeat movement until set is complete on one leg and then switch legs and repeat movement.

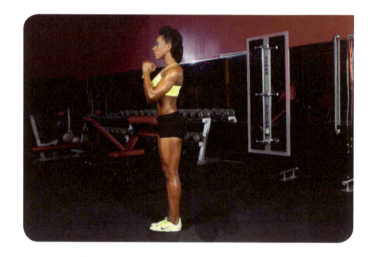

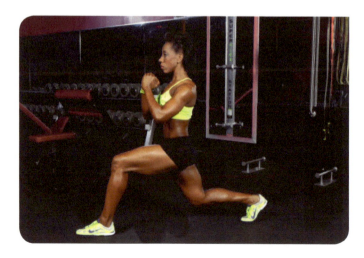

REVERSE LUNGE WITH ABDUCTIONS

Targeted Muscles: quadriceps, glutes and hamstrings

Set Up: Stand with feet together, slight bend in knees, shoulders back, core engaged with hands resting on hips.

Action: In a slow and controlled manner, step back with one leg, creating a wide stance between your front and back leg. Keep a slight bend in both knees without knees going over toes. Your back knee approaches the ground but never touches the ground. Once in this position, hold for a count and then bring back leg forward to starting position.

From starting position, place sight bend in lead leg and move your leg away from the midline (middle) of your body. Hold for a count and then bring leg back to starting position. Switch legs and repeat movements with opposite leg.

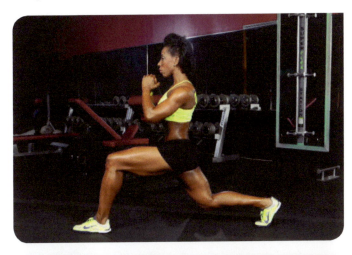

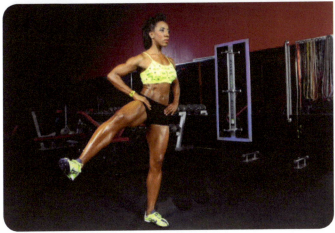

SQUAT WITH SIDE KICK

Targeted Muscles: Glutes, hamstrings

Set Up: Stand with feet hip width apart, core tight and shoulder blades retracted

Action: In a slow and controlled manner, engage core and squat until your knees make a 90 degree angle. Hold squat for a count while maintaining proper form. Return completely from squat, shift weight onto right leg, and then kick out to the left side of your body. Bring leg back to ground, repeat squatting movement and perform kick with opposite leg.

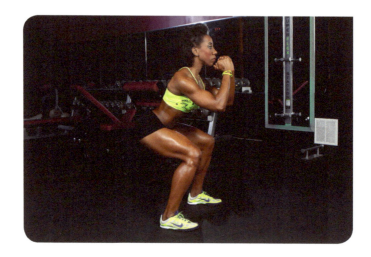

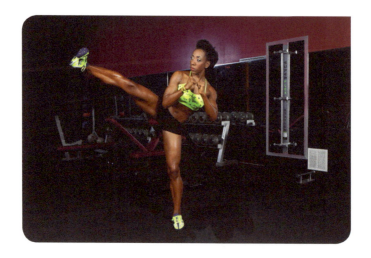

PLIE SQUATS WITH CALF RAISES

Targeted Muscles: calves, inner thighs, glutes

Set Up: Stand with feet wider than shoulder width apart, toes turned outward with core engaged and arms extended by body.

Action: In a slow and controlled manner, lower body until your thighs are parallel to the ground. Keep knees pointed in same direction as toes. Hold for a count and then return body back to starting position. While in an upward position, lift up on calves and perform a calve raise. Bring calves down. Repeat entire movement until set is complete.

*Movement Tip: Keep core contracted throughout entire movement. Do not allow knees to go over toes.

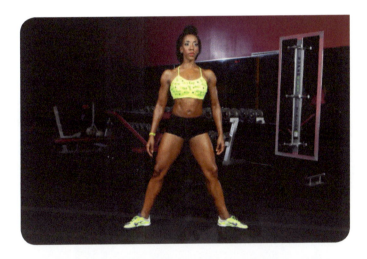

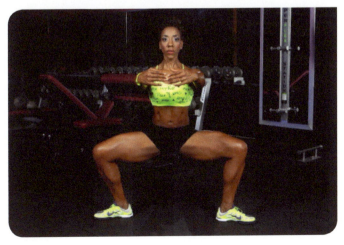

LATERAL LUNGES

Targeted Muscles: Glutes, hamstrings

Set Up: Place feet together or hip-width apart with your toes pointed directly forward. Shoulders back, core engaged and hands placed in front of body or positioned on hips.

Action: In a slow and controlled manner, lift your right leg and step to the side. Once your foot is fully planted, push your hips back and bend your right knee to lower into a lunge. Descend until your right thigh is about parallel to the floor and then extend your hips and knee to come back up.

Return your right foot to the starting position and then perform the next repetition, stepping to the side with your left foot. Continue this back and forth movement pattern until you complete set.

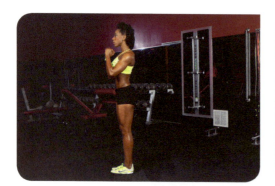
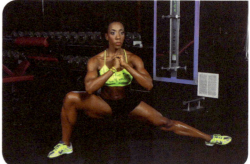
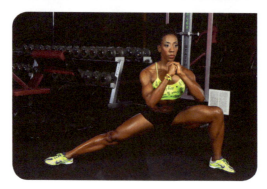

LUNGE UPS

Targeted Muscles: glutes, thighs (quadriceps) & hamstrings

Set Up: Begin with body in a stationary lunge position, right leg back, core engaged with hands positioned in front of body or on hips.

Action: In a slow and controlled manner, push off back leg, bringing body into an upward position shifting weight from back leg to front left leg. Hold body in this position for a count and then slowly lower right leg back to starting position. Repeat movement pattern on right leg until set is complete and then switch legs and repeat movement until set is complete.

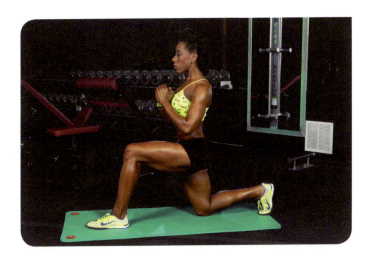

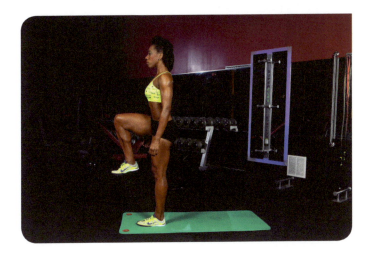

Targeted Muscle: glutes, hamstrings

Set Up: Lie on your back with both feet placed on the ground knees bent, with arms extended by your side.

Action: In a slow and controlled manner, slowly lift right leg off ground, while bridging up on left leg by squeezing your glutes and hamstrings. Hold body in this position for a count and then slowly lower left hip and right leg. Switch legs and repeat movement pattern on the opposite side of your body until set is complete.

*Modified Version: Keep both feet on ground, and then bridge up.

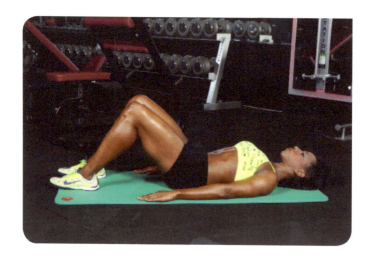

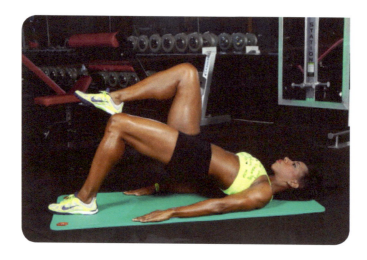

HAMSTRING REACH

Targeted Muscles: glutes, hamstrings

Set Up: Stand with feet together, slight bend in knees. Arms extended by your side with hands in a neutral position (palms facing inwards towards your body).

Action: While maintaining a slight bend in knees and core engaged, in a slow and controlled manner, bring torso forward reaching dumbbells towards ground and pushing hips back. Hold for a count and then return body back to starting position. Repeat movement until set is complete.

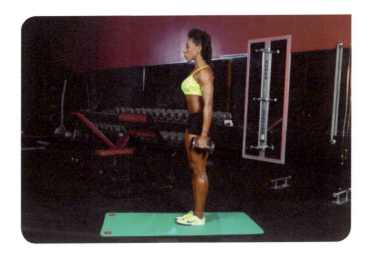

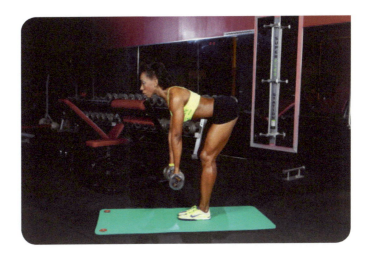

FROG LIFTS

Targeted Muscles: glutes, hamstrings

Set Up: Roll forward on stability ball until hips are positioned midway on ball, legs spread apart forming a "V," feet touching ground with arms positioned shoulder width apart.

Action: While keeping legs in "V" position, in a slow and controlled manner, squeeze glutes and move legs in an upward movement towards the ceiling. Hold for a count and then bring legs back to starting position. Repeat movement until set is complete.

*Movement Tip: Keep a slight bend in elbows throughout entire movement. Keep head forward in a neutral position.

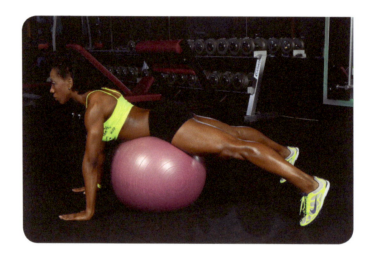

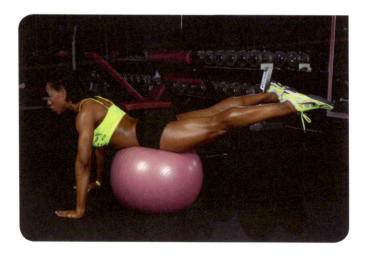

HAMSTRING BLAST

Targeted Muscles: hamstrings, glutes

Set Up: Lay on your back with knees bent, feet flat on stability ball, arms resting near body with palms in a downward position.

Action: In a slow and controlled manner, create an arc movement by pressing feet against ball and lifting hips off ground. Hold for a count and then return body back to starting position. Repeat movement until set is complete.

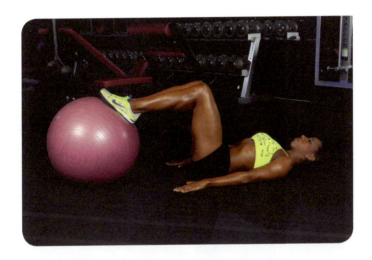

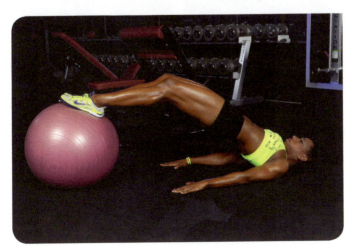

CURTSY LUNGE

Targeted Muscle: quads, glutes, hamstrings

Set Up: Stand with right leg in front and left leg positioned diagonally behind right leg. Slight bend in knees, with hands rested on hips.

Action: In a slow and controlled manner, bend both knees until your thigh is parallel to the ground. Your back knees approaches, but never touches the ground. Hold for a count and then return body back to starting position. Repeat movement until set is complete and then switch front and back legs, repeat movement with opposite stance until set is complete.

*Movement Tip: Make sure knee doesn't go past toes. Keep body in proper alignment with core contracted throughout entire movement.

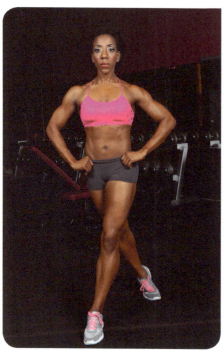 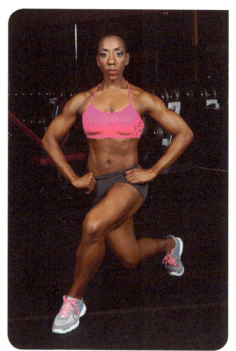

FIT JEWEL

You can't spot reduce to lose weight in a particular part of your legs! You can train smart, consistently and consume healthy well-balanced meals to assist you in losing weight in your legs and your entire body

TICK TOCKS

Targeted Muscle: glutes, quads (thighs) and hamstrings

Set Up: Stand with feet together, slight bend in knees, arms by your side.

Action: While contracting core, in a slow and controlled manner, bring torso forward reaching both arms in front of body while lifting right leg off the ground. Keep eyes forward and locate a focal point in order to maintain balance. Hold body in this position for a count and then bring body back to starting position. Repeat movement and switch legs. Repeat movement pattern until set is complete.

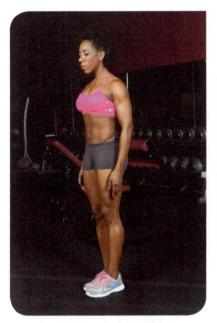
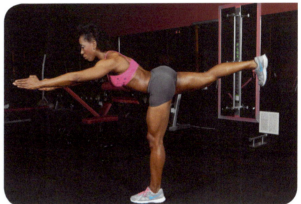

FIT JEWEL

Squat, lunge and bridge for tighter and firmer legs, but don't forget clean eating and regular cardio to help you shed unwanted body fat from your legs. Don't let your hard work go to waste!

STANDING HIP ABDUCTIONS

Targeted Muscles: abductors, glutes

Set Up: Stand with feet together, slight bend in knees. Hands placed on hips or in front of your body.

Action: With slight bend in knee, in a slow and controlled manner, lift leg off ground away from the mid-line or middle of body with knee pointing downward. Keep bend in opposite leg. Hold for a count and then return leg back to starting position. Repeat movement and then switch leg and repeat movement until set is complete with opposite leg.

***Movement Tip:** While lifting leg, keep core tight to avoid a shift of weight on supporting leg. If you lack balance or core strength, find an object to hold onto for support.

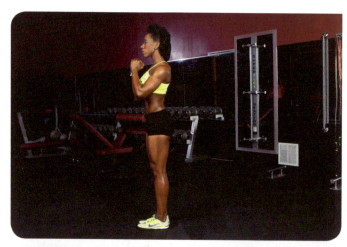

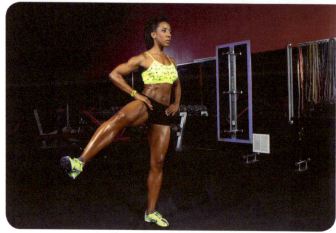

DEVELOPED GLUTES LOOK GREAT IN ANYTHING YOU WEAR!

Abdominal Exercises

Stronger Core! A Stronger You.

A Your core or abdominal muscles are one of the most important muscle groups in the entire body. Every movement performed requires core stabilization and strength. For some women, this is a challenging area to tone and strengthen. Some women have given birth and as a result have weakened core muscles. On the other hand, some women have jobs that require long hours of sitting and as a result, their core muscles have been weakened and they experience low back pain. Regardless of your profession or whether you are a mother, having a strong core is essential to all of your movements.

Therefore the exercises on the following pages will help you create a more toned and strong core.

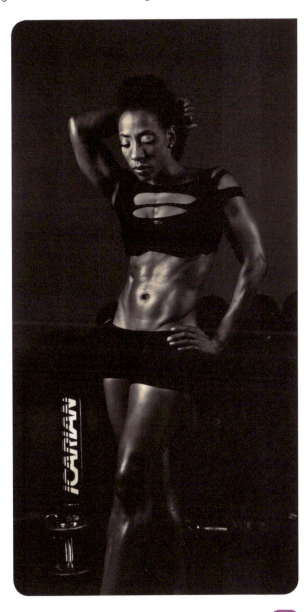

ABDOMINAL EXERCISES

Movement Tip: Keep core contracted while performing each exercise. This will keep body aligned and lessen the chance of injury to your back.

BEGINNER LEVEL

Exercise	Sets	Repetitions
Knee Taps	2	8-10
Physio-ball reverse knees	2	8-10
Ropes	2	8-10
Walk-Ups	2	8-10

INTERMEDIATE LEVEL

Exercise	Sets	Repetitions
Russian Twists with Layout	2-3	12-15
Med-ball Oblique Twists	2-3	12-15
Hanging Abdominal Raises	2-3	12-15
Ropes	2-3	12-15

ADVANCED LEVEL

Exercise	Sets	Repetitions
Russian Twists with Layout	3-4	15-20
Med-ball Oblique Twists	3-4	15-20
Hanging Abdominal Raises	3-4	15-20
Ropes	3-4	15-20

KNEE TAPS

Targeted Muscles: obliques

Set Up: Begin with feet placed shoulder width apart, slight bend in knees with arms extended overhead while holding medicine ball.

Action: In a slow and controlled manner, contract core and bring right elbow and right knee together, hold for a count. Return to starting position. Repeat movement until set is complete. Switch arm and leg and then repeat movement until set is complete.

*Movement Tip: Keep slight bend in knees throughout entire movement.

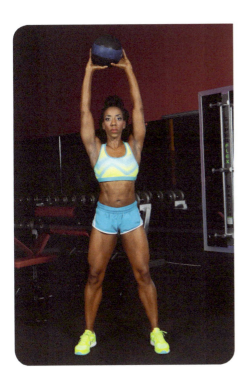
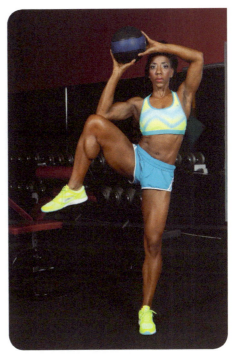

WALK-UPS

Targeted Muscles: abdominals

Set Up: Begin in a push up position, arms shoulder width apart with slight bend in elbows, core tight, lower body in a straight line.

Action: In a slow and controlled manner, step backwards with your hands until your body is in a "V" position. Hold position for a count and then slowly bring body down by moving hands forwards. Repeat movement until set is complete.

*Movement Tip: Only go as far as your natural range of motion will allow.

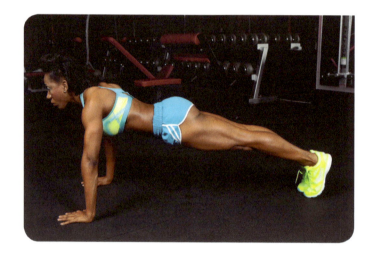

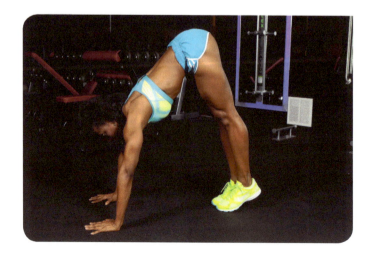

RUSSIAN TWISTS WITH LAYOUT

Targeted Muscles: abdominals, obliques

Set Up: Place body on mat with feet flat on ground, knees bent, chest up while arms are bent holding medicine ball.

Action: In a slow and controlled manner, bring feet off mat around 2-4 inches. Once stabilized, rotate torso from one side to the other side of the body. After rotation, return torso to starting position, while in this position extend arms overhead and release legs straight in front of your body. Hold for a count and then repeat movement until set is complete.

*Modified Version: Keep feet on ground when rotating and do not perform layout.

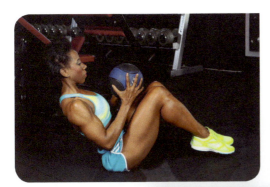 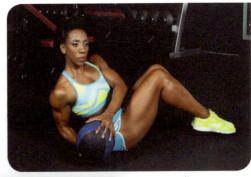

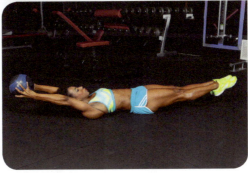

SWITCH-N-REACH

Targeted Muscles: obliques

Set Up: Lie down on a mat with body in a jumping jack position. Arms and legs form an "X".

Action: In a slow and controlled manner, bring right arm towards left leg. Hold for a count and then bring body back to staring position. From starting position, switch arm and leg and repeat movement until set is complete.

Movement Tip: Only lift arm and leg within natural range of motion.

*Modified Version: Keep upper body in same position with legs placed on ground. Instead of bringing arm and leg together, reach opposite arm towards opposite leg by slightly lifting shoulder off mat.

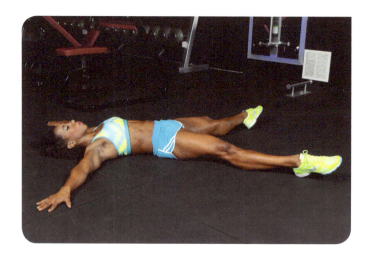

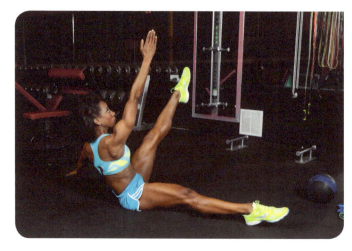

PIKE HOLDS

Targeted Muscles: abdominals

Set Up: In a slow and controlled manner, roll body forward on stability ball until shins rest on ball. Hands are positioned shoulder width apart, core tight and legs in a straight line.

Action: With a slight bend in elbows, in a slow and controlled manner, slowly draw in stomach and lift body into a pike position creating a "V." Hold for a count and then slowly bring body back to starting position. Repeat movement until set is complete.

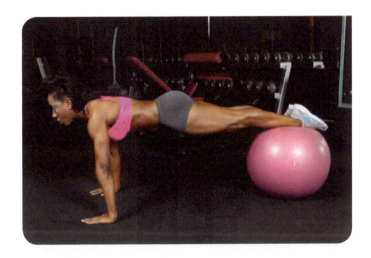

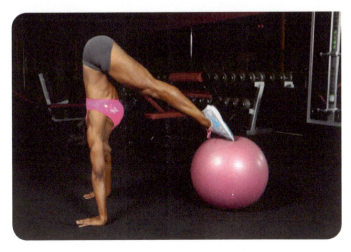

WINDMILLS

Targeted Muscles: abdominals, obliques

Set Up: While lying on your back, extend both arms out to the side of your body, with left leg fully extended and right knee bent with foot on floor.

Action: In a slow and controlled manner lift upper body off ground in a rotational movement, reaching left arms towards right knee, while right foot lifts off ground. Hold for a count and rotate body back to starting position. Perform movement until set is complete. Switch legs and repeat entire movement on opposite side.

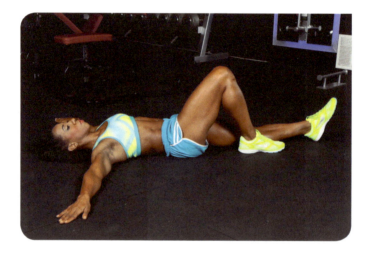

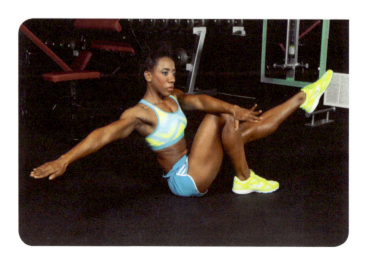

PHYSIO-BALL REVERSE KNEES

Targeted Muscles: abdominals

Set Up: While lying on your back, place physio-ball in between your legs, slightly squeezing your thigh muscles to keep the ball stabilized. Feet are at in a flexed position on ground.

Action: In a slow and controlled manner, engage core and bring feet off ground and knees towards upper body. Hold for a count and slowly bring feet back to ground without allowing feet to fully rest on ground. Repeat movement until set is completed.

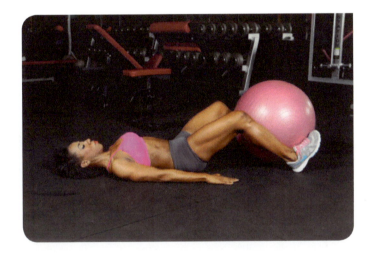

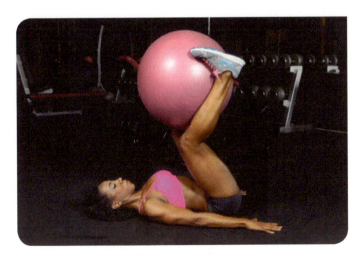

MED-BALL OBLIQUE TWISTS

Targeted Muscles: abdominals, obliques

Set up: While lying on your back, with arms extended on ground next to body, knees bent, place medicine ball between thigh muscles, with feet flat on ground.

Action: In a slow and controlled manner, lift feet off ground and rotate hips and knees towards the side of your body. Hold for a count and then bring legs back to the middle of your body and rotate them in the opposite direction and hold for a count. Repeat this movement pattern until set is complete.

Movement tip: Try to keep shoulders on ground when rotating body from side to side. If you can't properly execute movement with medicine ball, remove medicine ball and perform movement without it.

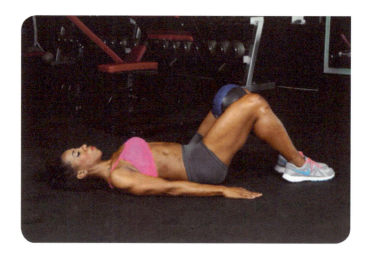

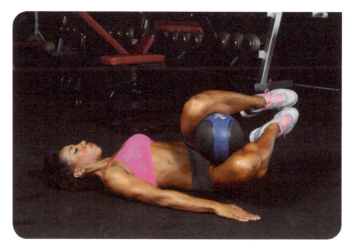

ROPES

Targeted Muscles: abdominals

Set Up: Lay on ground with knees bent, feet flat on floor and arms extended over your head, with one arm staggered over the other.

Action: In a slow and controlled manner engage your core and pretend your hands are climbing up a rope, one hand at a time. Once body is completely off the floor, hold for a count and then slowly reverse your hands climbing back down the rope as your torso returns back to the ground. Repeat movement until set is completed.

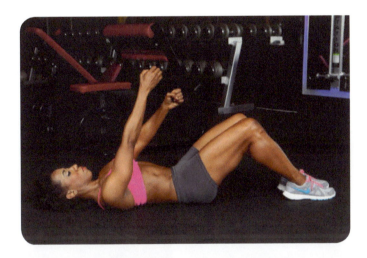

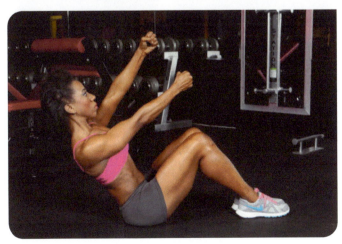

HANGING ABDOMINAL RAISES

Targeted Muscles: abdominals

Set Up: In a slow and controlled manner, jump up or use a bench to grasp and hang from a high bar (Universal Machine) with hands positioned slightly wider than shoulder width apart with and overhand grip, core engaged and body stabilized.

Action: In a slow and controlled manner, slowly raise legs by flexing hips and knees until hips are completely flexed or knees are well above hips. Hold for a count and then slowly return hips and knees to starting position. Repeat movement until set is completed.

Movement tip: When performing this movement do not allow body to swing back and forth. Keep core engaged throughout entire movement and keep slight bend in elbows while hanging from bar.

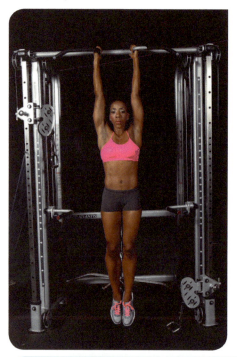 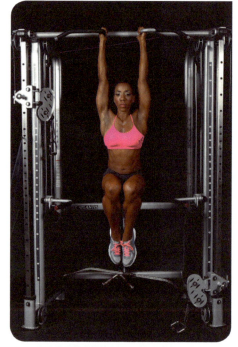

FIT JEWEL

Don't focus solely on getting a 4 or 6 pack. Instead focus on building a strong core that will support your body for the rest of your life!

CURVE SCULPTING EXERCISE TRACKING SHEET

USE THE FOLLOWING sheet to track your exercises, rank intensity levels and mental preparedness for each workout.

Make copies of this sheet and place into a binder to create your own fitness training log.

Date:			
Exercise	**Sets**	**Repitions**	**Rest Time**
Mental Fit:			

Having a positive attitude about your workout can produce great results. Therefore, before you start your workout, take time to gauge your mental preparation.

Rank your mindset for your workout:

1. I am extremely focused.
2. I am tired, but no more excuses.
3. I will do it because I have to.
4. I am excited about seeing my body change.

Intensity Level:

The amount of effort you put into your workout will determine your overall results.

Rank the amount of effort you put into your workout.

1. I gave 100% - no slacking.
2. I could have pushed harder.
3. I wasn't excited about the workout, but gave it all I had.

145

YOU ROCK!

As you end with this chapter, I am very excited to know that you have the tools to transform your body. Remember, let go of all the myths about women and weight training and work on being the fittest vesion of yourself. Not a fit version of your girlfriend or the lady on the fitness magazine cover, work on getting into the best shape of your life, for YOURSELF on YOUR terms! You've learned a lot of great information in this book that when applied works and can result in amazing improvements to your overall conditioning and fitness level.

I am 100% sure of this statement. The information you have read is evidence-based and scientific. Don't get overwhelmed with applying everything you've learned in short period of time, rather take your time and enjoy the process!

I've been doing this for over 15 years and still love every moment of it, but I didn't learn everything overnigght!

In closing, here's to you feeling FIT, INSPIRED and EMPOWERED!

Bye the way, did I tell you that you ROCK?

This isn't good-bye, because I look forward to hearing what you have discovered about yourself, and how you are transforming your body!

Therefore please e-mail me and share your personal story at laticiamariejackson@gmail.com.

LATICIA "ACTION" JACKSON - STAY FIT, STAY TRUE, STAY YOU!

IFBB Fitness Pro/Fitness Expert

3-Time N.P.C. Fitness Champion

2008 Fitness Olympian

ABOUT THE AUTHOR

LATICIA " ACTION" JACKSON

LIFESTYLE AND FITNESS Expert Laticia "Action" Jackson has been recognized as one of the most energetic and passionate personalities in the health promotion, wellness and fitness industry. She brings to these fields over 15 years of combined experience.

She holds a Master's Degree in Public Health, B.S. Degree in Exercise Science, A.A. Degree in Human Performance, Certified Personal Trainer, Certified Lifestyle and Weight Management Specialists and Certified Weight Loss Counselor.

She's a 3-Time N.P.C. (National Physique Committee) National Fitness Champion and 2008 Fitness Olympian. She has been featured in over 11 nationally-recognized fit-

ness publications (Oxygen, Muscle and Fitness Hers, Flex, Ironman, Muscular Development) and has made multiple television appearances for stations such as Fox 45/ABC 22 and C.W. 31 as the go-to fitness expert.

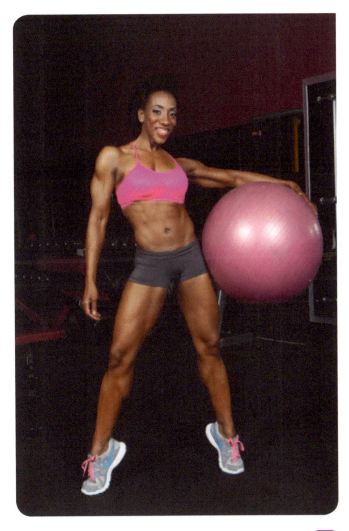

As a survivor of domestic violence, it has become her mission to encourage women to love themselves by providing them with the tools to become fit from the inside out. As a Veteran of the U.S.A.F., her discipline and determination has catapulted her fitness and educational career to great heights. She is a member of Delta Sigma Theta Sorority and enjoys volunteering and giving back to her community.

Index

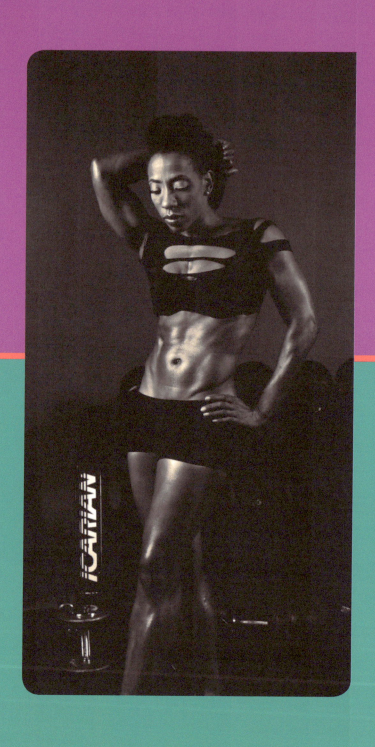

YES WOMEN LIFT!

A WOMAN'S GUIDE TO LIFTING WEIGHTS AND FEELING GREAT

LATICIA "ACTION" JACKSON

CPSIA information can be obtained
at www.ICGtesting.com
Printed in the USA
LVHW02n2334070618
580048LV00005B/23/P

9 781545 360408